UNBREAKABLE RUNNER

UNBREAKABLE RUNNER

Unleash the power of strength & conditioning for a lifetime of running strong

T.J. Murphy & Brian MacKenzie

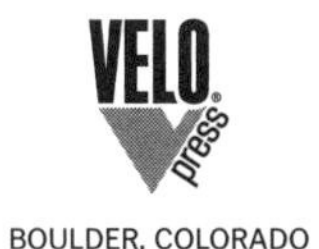

BOULDER, COLORADO

This book is intended as a reference only. The information it contains is designed to help you make informed decisions about your own health and fitness programs. It is not intended as a substitute for professional medical or fitness advice. As with all exercise programs, you should seek your doctor's approval before you begin.

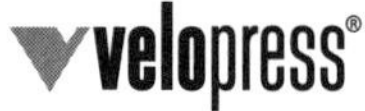

3002 Sterling Circle, Suite 100
Boulder, Colorado 80301-2338 USA
(303) 440-0601 · Fax (303) 444-6788 · E-mail velopress@competitorgroup.com

Distributed in the United States and Canada by Ingram Publisher Services

A Cataloging-in-Publication record for this book is available from the Library of Congress.
ISBN 978-1-937715-14-4

For information on purchasing VeloPress books, please call (800) 811-4210, ext. 2138, or visit www.velopress.com.

This paper meets the requirements of ANSI/NISO Z39.48-1992 (Permanence of Paper).

Cover design by Scott Erwert
Cover photograph, exercise photographs in Chapter 5, and Brian MacKenzie author photograph, page 211, by Christopher Bishow
T.J. Murphy author photograph, page 211, by Scott Draper
Interior design by Anita Koury

Text set in Poynter

14 15 16 / 10 9 8 7 6 5 4 3 2 1

Dedicated to Kelly Starrett; Barry Sears; Nicholas Romanov; and especially my coauthor, Brian MacKenzie, whose steadfast courage in applying clear thought and experimentation to solve old, deep-rooted problems is as inspiring as it is appreciated.

—T.J. Murphy

I dedicate this to every athlete, every coach, and every person who has reminded me that change and an open mind are the only way we advance anything. It is with great conviction that I know this is not the only way to train. My only purpose has been to be a messenger and to tell the truth about what we've learned.

Forever a student.

—Brian MacKenzie

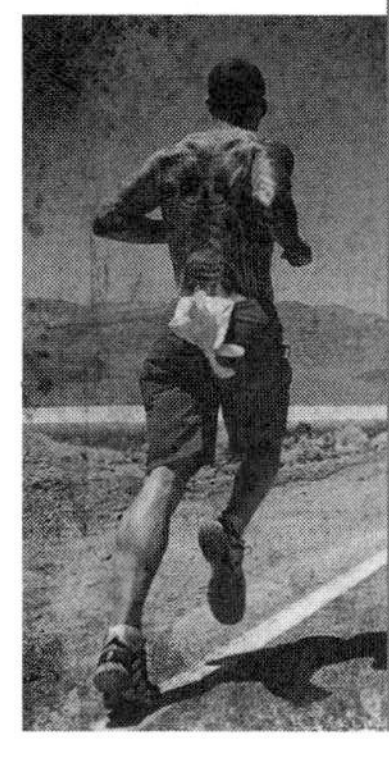

CONTENTS

FOREWORD

In my home office, I keep a file cabinet and bookshelf that together serve as a central repository for what I consider indispensable information regarding my running and athletic performance. It's a sacred place where I catalog the various books, reports, and studies meticulously gathered from the world of sports science. As my wife described in a chapter she authored in my book *Run!*, I can get pretty swept away in detailing the nutrition and gear strategies that go into an obstacle race or a run across the continent. I love it all—it's what I live for.

This storehouse of information represents my passion for being a student of the vast amount of work that goes into the "before" part of racing and preparing the body—and the mind—for the rigors of endurance competition. How can I fine-tune my diet toward optimal health? How can I use strength training to maximize performance and prevent injury? What can I do to improve my running form and efficiency? What is the best way to train for varying distances and varying conditions? What sort of gear and acclimatization strategy are optimal for the subzero cold of the South Pole or the blazing heat of Death Valley?

The reward comes on days when things flow perfectly, when the miles unfold in sync and all goes smoothly and according to plan.

But perhaps an even more valuable payoff for my obsession with the ancillary topics related to human performance comes on those days when things *don't* go according to plan—such as when your body starts rebelling in the first 30 miles of a 3,000-mile Run Across America. That's when you really learn about what your body needs, whether it's a particular kind of food, a more targeted hydration and electrolyte replenishment plan, or improved stability and strength. With each problem that arises, I think back to the data I've collected, and I try to recall the relevant advice and information that I've read. Much of my success in running has been due to my ability to apply this information to get back on track.

My passion for absorbing as much knowledge as possible about the art and science of distance running has, without a doubt, been crucial to an increasingly long, injury-free ultrarunning career. In a sport widely known as a pursuit in which feet, knees, and hips routinely get chewed up, my record is something of an oddity. I've been able to keep running mile after mile without issues, and I credit my willingness to sometimes do things differently, to experiment with training, in order to get the absolute best out of myself.

To some people I might seem obsessive, but there are others who share my passion for understanding the act of running and for constantly seeking to improve. Brian MacKenzie is one of these. For a new generation of runners around the world who have taken up CrossFit and CrossFit Endurance, Brian has been a godsend. His hunger for knowledge has been insatiable since he himself started "chasing the dragon," as he likes to call the beast that is long-course endurance racing. Whether he's competing in ultramarathons or Ironman® triathlons, Brian has feverishly tinkered with the many variables that go into the craft, from diet to minimalist footwear to the use of strength conditioning as a way both to improve performance and to ward off injury.

Brian's strategies and coaching methods are employed at CrossFit gyms and other training facilities across the planet. His rigorous process of testing and evaluating new ideas, and interesting combinations of new ideas, has opened doors to coaches and runners, offering proven solutions to a myriad of problems that persistently vex runners of all ages, abilities, and backgrounds.

Thanks to the pioneering work of mavericks like Brian, the running world is increasingly tuning in to the merits of high-intensity strength training and progressively making diet and nutrition central components of an athlete's overall life. The image of the distance runner as a lone figure who simply logs tons of miles while carbo-loading truckloads of pasta is fading fast. The world has progressed.

This book represents Brian's current thinking on how best to become an unbreakable runner. And don't we all want to be that? It is a valuable tool that is now indispensable on my bookshelf and has helped me immeasurably in my preparation for the next adventure.

May the journey never end!

—DEAN KARNAZES

New York Times *best-selling author-athlete Dean Karnazes once ran 50 marathons in all 50 states in 50 consecutive days. Named by* Time *magazine one of the "Top 100 Most Influential People on Earth," Dean lives with his wife and family in the San Francisco Bay Area.*

WRITER'S NOTE

The first time Brian MacKenzie and I corresponded, it wasn't pretty. We wanted to kill each other.

I was editor in chief of *Triathlete* magazine, and I had a freelance writer working on a story about MacKenzie and the controversial training program he had founded, CrossFit Endurance (CFE). Depending on whom you listened to, it was either the best training innovation since the interval workout or a fatal virus out to destroy all that was pure and good in running.

As I started to sense how polarizing MacKenzie and the program were, I took a few steps back. In the magazine world, more complicated stories sometimes get pushed to a later issue, or they sometimes get killed completely and never run. We decided to push this story to a later issue so we could take our time with it. Wires got crossed, and although I had only delayed the story, it was MacKenzie's understanding that I'd killed it.

MacKenzie went ballistic. He sent out a social media call to arms, recruiting the growing community of runners and triathletes who swore by his training principles with religious intensity. On his blog,

MacKenzie posted his grievance along with my e-mail address and asked readers to let me know what they thought about my killing the story. E-mails tumbled into my in-box as if I'd just won at slots. Some were diplomatic, asking me to reconsider the decision not to publish a story on CFE. Others were borderline violent.

I contacted MacKenzie and asked with undisguised incredulity, "What is your problem?"

It took a while to sort out what had happened. But for the better part of a day, we wanted to kill each other.

To be fair, MacKenzie's defensiveness wasn't difficult to understand. CrossFit Endurance—and he along with it—had been vilified in popular running and triathlon online forums. Some of the discussions were vitriolic. In one instance, he was dubbed "the Antichrist."

It's not hard to understand the critics' side, either. Then, as now, MacKenzie's training methods and his program openly challenged some of the very foundations of distance running theory. Within the competitive distance running culture, honest, hard work is the metric by which a runner is often judged, and to some, at first glance, CFE can appear to be a cheap shortcut to success. To others, it seems dead wrong and even dangerous. After all, CFE is at odds with just about every sacred cow in running, including notions about how much to run, what to eat, whether or not a runner should lift weights, what kind of shoes to wear, ideas about stretching, and the use of periodization.

For example, in his lecture videos, MacKenzie discusses the negative consequences of too much mileage. In one, he talks about how too much running volume can increase the speed of aging through the production of free radicals and the subsequent effects of oxidation. The result is an endurance athlete wrinkled beyond his or her years. In the lecture, he says that he, too, has suffered such effects from his early days of running big miles.

When I first saw these videos, I was as offended as any traditionalist. Who was this guy with tattoos on his arms and knuckles, associated with some flavor-of-the-month fitness cult, to cast arrows at the methods followed by our modern heroes of endurance athletics? Outraged, but admittedly a little intrigued by his audacity, I wanted to know the whole story. So I first assigned the story to a freelancer with knowledge of the CrossFit world, something I didn't possess.

However, after the electronic ambush from MacKenzie's posse and my own confrontation with MacKenzie, I decided to write the story myself. Truly sweeping and new ideas in endurance training don't come along that often. Just about every training philosophy I was aware of was a variation on the same old plan: Build a big aerobic base, then add in the strength and speed work, and then race. To write about an approach that turned that model inside out would be invigorating. And if it really was just a get-rich-quick scheme, I wanted to be the one to debunk it.

But what happened to me next was unexpected. I continued watching MacKenzie's CFE lecture videos as he ticked through the long-held tenets of distance running, such as doing high mileage, focusing on long runs, and incorporating periodization. He systematically rejected them all, supplanting them with priorities such as skill work, strength and conditioning, and replacing cardiovascular endurance with muscular stamina. I flinched with each swap, but I kept listening, and in each case, I found I had a hard time refuting his argument.

In one lecture, MacKenzie spoke about how members of the traditional endurance community who had once vowed to never set foot in his gym "come in, their heads lowered, ready to try it." MacKenzie explains this is because "they're tired of being beat to shit."

Cue my temper. No one shall insult the high-mileage ethic while on my watch. But then I took a few minutes to think about it. Unfortunately, I myself was a shining example of why MacKenzie might have a point. Here I was, a limping mess of a former runner who had recently been unable even to complete one of the vaunted high-mileage programs I so fiercely advocated. A thick ring of calcium had grown around the connective tissue attached to my left heel bone. My right thigh had atrophied, likely because the cartilage in my right knee resembled Swiss cheese and provided little support to the surrounding muscle. My left hamstring contained a marble-sized knot of scar tissue, and my lower back had been prone to complete blowouts. I was a broken runner.

But it hadn't started out that way. I had found early success with traditional high-mileage training schedules. My progress quickly peaked, however, then receded. Between 1994 and 2011, I spent more and more of my time unable to run a step. Instead, I was icing, sitting atop a Lifecycle or aqua jogging, and calculating how many Advil I could safely take in a day. I no longer thought of running as being enjoyable, and I went through several long spells where I could no longer honestly consider myself a runner at all.

MacKenzie talked about runners who, like me, were broken but went through his program and were restored. Digging deeper for that *Triathlete* magazine piece, I interviewed a triathlete who had been hit by a car, sustaining injuries for which his doctor predicted a long, slow road to recovery. He started a CFE program and within a single summer was achieving new personal best running times.

I interviewed another triathlete who had left behind conventional high-volume Ironman training for CFE. She told me that during a routine visit to her physical therapist, the PT was shocked at how much her alignment, balance, and mobility had improved. "Whatever it is you're doing, keep doing it," the therapist told her.

In contrast, with my limp, trick back, and increasing body fat percentage, I would have made a vivid exhibit for MacKenzie and his coaches to cart along to their lectures to show what can eventually happen to mileage addicts. I was a little like the guy with a tracheotomy whom you would bring to an antismoking talk for kids: "See, gang, you can get away with some of these fundamental errors you've been making in your training, but one day you'll end up like this guy."

I decided to give CFE a try. What did I have to lose? If it meant risking an injury, it didn't seem like much of a risk, given what I was already dealing with.

Around that time, MacKenzie happened to be holding a CFE seminar in San Diego, where I lived and worked. I drove up to visit. I parked at the side of the building, gingerly pried myself out of my car, as usual, and took 50 yards to loosen up so I could hide my limp as much as possible.

I found MacKenzie in a room with a group of students, reviewing a videotape of their running. His passion was palpable. As he reviewed the video, he was animated, articulate, and impassioned in his analysis and prescriptions. He was a coach on a mission.

At a break in the seminar, MacKenzie and I talked in person for the first time. Since that day, I've written about CFE and Brian MacKenzie many times. I've called him with questions about some of the most specific nuances of running and triathlon, and he's never failed to give me an answer that was both rich and illuminating. This led to a major personal overhaul of my training and racing that I detailed in my first book, *Inside the Box*.

It's not an exaggeration to say that the journey I began with MacKenzie has changed my running life. It has also created within me the same kind of passion that MacKenzie has for sharing this powerful method with other runners.

It's my hope that the information contained in this book will help you reach all of your running goals, whatever they may be, and keep you running for life.

—T.J. MURPHY

INTRODUCTION
A NEW WAY UP TO THE MOUNTAINTOP

Nearly every coaching plan available in the running world today is an iteration of a model developed by famed New Zealand coach Arthur Lydiard (1917–2004).

Lydiard's runners spent at least 8 weeks—often more—building an aerobic base. The essential tool for building this base was the standard training run. Although many training plans refer to this workout by the acronym "LSD" (for long, slow distance), Lydiard did not intend these to be easy jogs; he intended them to be up-tempo strength runs. But whether you were an 800-meter runner or a long-distance athlete, you ran at least 100 miles per week during this 8-week period, punctuated by a weekly long run of 20 miles or more.

Following this base-building phase came a month of hill work during which runners used a form Lydiard called "springing." This was a kind of bounding that prepared runners for the speed phases of the program. After 4 weeks of hill training, Lydiard's runners moved on to traditional speed work, running intervals on a track, followed by a peaking period that was intended to bring them to their best possible performance.

Lydiard's method won his runners six gold medals in the 1960 Olympics and ignited what would become the Lydiard era. He spent the following decades establishing his philosophy in countries such as Finland, Japan, and Mexico, each of which had its day as a world-beater. Where Lydiard went, gold medals followed.

So in 1989, at age 26, when I decided to try a marathon, I naturally decided to train the Lydiard way.

The CFE program is about two words you do not hear much about in traditional programs: health and sustainability.

I used a derivative plan that included a base-building phase, a hill phase, and a speed phase. The plan prescribed a long run every other week, which slowly increased to more than 20 miles. The speed phase included a session of mile repeats, peaking with a total of more than 10 × 1 mile for a single workout.

The program was, I had to admit, pretty boring, especially the track work. I spent a lot of time going around in circles. But the method worked for me. I ran my first marathon in 3:24, my second in 2:52, my third in 2:49, and my fourth in 2:38.

This success cemented my belief in the Lydiard model of training. Unfortunately, though, that success was not long-lived. After my fourth marathon, I started to find myself dealing with injuries between occasional bouts of successful running. Still, I remained a staunch disciple and defender of Lydiard and the high-mileage work ethic, for which author John L. Parker coined the phrase "the Trial of Miles."

For years I kept trying to regain the ability to carry out the Trial of Miles. I added core training, chiropractic and physical therapy, stretching, icing, and anti-inflammatories to my program but gained only minimal relief from injuries. Yet somehow I didn't see a problem with what I was doing; injury was just a necessary hardship to be accepted along with the success.

After meeting Brian MacKenzie and listening to what he had to say, I started to rethink my loyalty to the Trial of Miles. The more I listened, the more I found that MacKenzie was not some ill-informed guru with eccentric beliefs about training that had no relevance for or connection with the "real" running world. Rather, he was thinking hard about and discussing the running community's core topics, from volume to health, running form, diet, and stretching. As a journalist, I quickly saw how this information—the monumental paradigm shifts taking place in the ideas behind run training—could be valuable to many readers, and a book project began to take shape in my mind.

MacKenzie, meanwhile, was frustrated by the tremendous gap between what he was teaching and what he was perceived to be teaching by much of the outside world. Part of the problem seemed to stem from the failure of many critics to differentiate between CrossFit, a general fitness program, and CrossFit Endurance (CFE), MacKenzie's sport-specific program that has CrossFit-style workouts as one of its pillars but is also much more.

For some critics, the mere presence of CrossFit strength workouts within a run-training program raises concerns. But MacKenzie is not the first coach to encourage runners to add elements such as lifting weights and performing high-intensity circuit work to their training. Nor is he the first coach to advocate gymnastics training for runners or to emphasize speed endurance over high mileage. In the 1950s and 1960s, Percy Cerutty—coach of Olympic gold medalist Herb Elliott—

embedded gymnastics and weight training in his training program. In the 1980s, Peter Coe—coach of Olympic gold medalist Sebastian Coe—rejected high-mileage theory in favor of heretical principles bound to speed endurance and circuit training.

Other critics complain that MacKenzie's program hasn't achieved Olympic success in the way that Lydiard's method has. The criticism is not inaccurate; however, it is also not a fair way to judge the program because MacKenzie's focus has been not on elite runners but rather on the mass of runners of average ability. These are athletes who run for the love of it, perhaps wanting to pursue better health or enjoy racing but with time restrictions that come with having a job or a family. MacKenzie tried to figure out how these runners could boost performance and still enjoy a lifelong, injury-free running career.

The final frustration for MacKenzie came when a 2012 *Outside* magazine story on him included a basic CrossFit Endurance training schedule. It was misunderstood by some readers to be a marathon training plan. This confusion reinvigorated CFE naysayers, launching a fresh Twitter attack.

Before long, MacKenzie and I decided to combine our complementary projects into one book. I would examine the foundational mechanics of MacKenzie's program from the point of view of a traditional runner who has spent time studying and using it. MacKenzie would produce training plans for the essential racing distances, illustrating how an athlete puts CFE theory into practice to prepare for an event.

What Is CrossFit Endurance?

As mentioned, MacKenzie works hard to overcome assumptions that some people make about CrossFit Endurance—such as that it is a bodybuilding routine, or that it is dangerous. Sometimes they simply aren't sure what difference exists between CrossFit and CFE. So for starters, what exactly is CrossFit Endurance?

CrossFit is a strength and conditioning program created by Greg Glassman. As defined by Glassman in the *CrossFit Journal*, CrossFit consists of "constantly varied functional movements executed at high intensity across broad time and modal domains." Consider the person who goes to a gym three times a week and performs the same 25-minute circuit of machines that isolate specific muscle groups, completing 2 sets of 10 reps for each exercise. Rest breaks occur between each exercise and set, rendering the workout low in terms of intensity. He or she does this every week, year after year, using the same machines, like the quad extension machine and the biceps curl machine, and always in the same order.

CrossFit is the polar opposite. Rather than using machines that isolate a muscle, CrossFit uses compound functional[1] exercises, such as burpees, that recruit a swath of muscle groups. Workouts constantly vary: What you do this Tuesday will be vastly different than what you did the previous Tuesday. Workout lengths range from a couple of minutes to 7 to 20 minutes; only rarely do they last 20 minutes or longer. There are no rest breaks. If it's a 10-minute workout consisting of push-ups, running intervals, and power cleans, then you move from set to set as quickly as possible. This mixture of compound movements with little or no rest ratchets up the intensity.

Along with an emphasis on healthy eating, that is the basic CrossFit program. The most important thing to know about CrossFit is that it is intended to develop high levels of fitness and health and an all-around athleticism. It's *not* sport-specific.

CrossFit Endurance, however, *is* sport-specific. A CFE running program, as Brian MacKenzie has developed it, prepares a runner for a race by combining specific running workouts, strength workouts, and CrossFit metabolic conditioning workouts. As MacKenzie asserts, the use of CrossFit workouts—with their myriad health and athletic benefits—allows a runner to obtain equal if not greater performance results while simultaneously decreasing the chance of injury.

So what results can CFE runners hope for? Under the CFE method, they can expect the following:

- Sustained or improved performance while running fewer miles overall
- Reduced injury risk as "junk" mileage is replaced with functional fitness workouts that train the same energy systems
- Increased explosive power and speed
- Less damage to mobility and range of motion through incorporating workouts that improve range of motion in the joints and muscle tissues
- Increased production of human growth hormone, which helps counter the natural loss of muscle mass that comes with age
- Revved-up fat-burning metabolism to burn excess body fat
- Improved coordination of upper- and lower-body muscle groups through the inclusion of compound movements in training
- Better race performance through greater strength, improved form, and greater running efficiency

All that probably sounds pretty good to you—maybe even a bit *too* good. Is there proof that CFE can deliver results? We will discuss some of these effects in later chapters, but first, let's take a closer look at training with intensity.

How Is This Possible?

As discussed earlier, most long-distance training plans adopt the standard Lydiard-based training model, which has high mileage as its cornerstone—the more miles, the better. There's no disputing that Lydiard developed a pathway for success, which he described in detail in his book *Running to the Top*. But is the high-mileage model the only way to the top? Or the healthiest?

Lydiard argued vehemently that it was, but not everyone agrees. For some, the risk of injury is not worth the benefits that high mileage bestows. For these runners, it makes more sense to make every step count than to take as many steps as possible.

Challenges to the Lydiard method did not start with MacKenzie. One of the first came in the 1980s from coach Peter Coe, who adopted a type of high-intensity interval training (HIIT) for his son, middle-distance runner Sebastian Coe. Their plan kept Seb's total mileage under 50 miles per week and included fast 200-meter repeats with 30 seconds of recovery between the fast segments. They also included weight training movements and plyometric exercises in a routine that looked similar to the typical CrossFit workouts one might see in a gym today.

How did this renegade training method work out for Seb? He won four Olympic gold medals in the 1980s, including gold in the 1500 meters in both 1980 and 1984. He set eight outdoor and three indoor world records in middle-distance track events—including, in 1979, setting three world records in the space of 41 days. The world record he set in the 800 meters in 1981 remained unbroken until 1997.

Even Lydiard would have had to admit that this method worked out pretty well for Seb, despite his relatively light mileage totals.

The HIIT approach has gone under the microscope as well, with scientists examining its influence on athletic performance. In a 1996 study, Izumi Tabata and his team tested the effects on athletes of 20 seconds of ultra-intense cycling followed by 10 seconds of rest, repeated 8 times, for a total testing time of about 4 minutes. Athletes using this method performed four 4-minute workouts per week and added another day of steady-state, lower-intensity cycling.

By the end of the study, the athletes using the HIIT method had obtained gains similar to those seen in a group of athletes who did only steady-state training, 5 times per week. While the steady-state group had a higher VO_2max[2] at the end, the HIIT group had started lower and gained more overall. These findings suggest that had all the athletes started at the same level, the HIIT-oriented group would have ended up with higher VO_2max scores. Also, only the Tabata group had gained anaerobic capacity benefits—meaning they had added not just endurance but also strength.[3]

A 2009 study by Martin Gibala and a team at McMaster University in Canada also took a close look at HIIT. Their study on students incorporated a 3-minute warm-up, followed by 60 seconds of intense exercise and 75 seconds of rest, repeated for 8 to 12 cycles. The total workout time ranged from 20 to 29 minutes, with the students repeating the routine 3 times per week for 2 weeks.

By the end of the testing period, subjects using this method obtained similar adaptations to the control group that used a "much larger volume of traditional endurance training." As the Gibala team concluded, "Given the markedly lower training volume in the sprint-interval group, these data suggest that high-intensity interval training is a time-efficient strategy to increase skeletal muscle oxidative capacity and induce specific metabolic adaptations during exercise that are comparable to traditional endurance training."[4]

In other words, with HIIT, you can get the same results as with high-volume training, but with less training.

These examples illustrate a central idea behind MacKenzie's program, which trades long aerobic runs for short, hard bouts of effort. But there is more to the CFE approach.

CrossFit Endurance is not limited to incorporating HIIT-based training principles, although that is central to the program. The CFE approach takes a much broader view of fitness than did Lydiard, or even Peter Coe. At its core, the CFE program is about two words you do not hear much about in traditional programs: health and sustainability.

As you'll discover in later chapters, a CFE athlete does not just run; he or she also works on developing running skill, balance, and flexibility. A CFE athlete also focuses on nutrition and mobility.

Why? Because ultimately, a CFE athlete is not just someone who runs and races well; he or she is someone who is, first and foremost, healthy and strong. As a result, a CFE athlete can also run very well and continue to do so injury-free.

Does CFE Work for Long-Distance Runners?

At this point, you might be convinced that a CFE approach may work for short- and middle-distance runners, but perhaps you wonder if it would work for longer distances. Can CFE really help marathoners? Or ultramarathoners? Those distances attract an almost reverential appreciation for repetitive motion and long training runs. How can a long-distance runner avoid running long distances and still expect to race strong?

The case for applying CFE principles to long-distance training and racing is actually even more compelling. In fact, the longer the distance, the more sense CFE makes.

The reason is the catch-22 that long-distance runners often face: the idea that to become a better runner, you need to run. A lot. But the more you run, the more likely you are to get injured and not be able to run.

The legendary running coach Jack Daniels has long counseled caution when it comes to high-mileage training. Daniels, who has been studying middle- and long-distance runners since the 1960s, recently conducted a survey of the first generation of runners that he took notes about. In 1968, as part of his dissertation research, Daniels had tested 26 elite long-distance runners. He retested the entire group in 1993 and tested it again in 2013. What results did Daniels find?

"Those that are the healthiest and fittest today," he says, "are the ones who missed the most days of running over the past decades."

In talks, Daniels often poses the following hypothetical question to a room full of runners: Consider two different training paths, one that requires 30 miles per week of training and another that requires 60 miles per week. Both will get you to a sub-5-minute mile. Which method would you pick?

For Daniels, the obvious choice is the plan with lower mileage. "Why would you pick 60 miles per week if you can accomplish the goal with 30? That'd be stupid," he says. "Do the least amount of work to get the maximum benefit."

Nevertheless, many of the runners to whom Daniels speaks prefer the option with more mileage. Why? Perhaps it's because of the deeply held historical regard for how high mileage leads to marathon excellence.

There is the impressive Lydiard medal count, detailed above. In the 1970s, when runners such as Frank Shorter and Bill Rodgers emerged as the greats during the first running boom, both were known for triple-digit weekly mileage levels. A decade earlier, Buddy Edelen ran 140 miles per week during training and set the world record in the marathon in 1963, logging a 2:14:28.

The rationale behind this training method wasn't just anecdotal. It was based on a highly regarded principle called the "rule of specificity." Under this dictum, the only way to become better at a given activity is to practice that activity.

The rule of specificity has often been cited to support the idea that runners should spend their training time running rather than on other forms of exercise. To get better, runners have to run. Period.

But while this approach has provided us with some great elite performances and new world records, it has also resulted in rampant injuries among those same runners as well as among the nonelites who try to emulate them. This seems like a high—and frustrating—price to pay.

Is CrossFit Endurance for You?

Is MacKenzie's way the only way to train? Certainly not. Although MacKenzie has been accused of preaching that his method is "the one true way" and that all elite athletes should be training like this, I've never heard him make such a sweeping declaration. In fact, the line he uses at seminars expresses quite the opposite: "There's more than one path to the mountaintop."

What MacKenzie is offering is an alternative. Yes, it is an alternative that he believes in fiercely, since it brought him back to health after his own high-mileage ultrarunning days left him beaten and destroyed. But he does not suggest it is the only path. Rather, the CFE model presents an alternative method of training that is useful for a broad range of runners.

First, it is for runners who find themselves in the situation both MacKenzie and I were in: the disheartening cycle of the endlessly injured. According to a Harvard study from 2012,[5] 79 percent of runners deal with an injury each year. And with nearly 10 million Americans running more than 110 days per year,[6] three out of four injured means a whole lot of damaged runners, many seeking help—and forking over lots of cash—in sports medicine clinics.

CrossFit Endurance offers an empowering alternative to that unpleasant roller coaster of success, then injury. First, it is a training program that requires less time and less pounding on the pavement, reducing the chance of injury. More important, it is the means to building and sustaining overall good health.

Prioritizing heath is the centerpiece of MacKenzie's CFE program. He believes not only that this is the right goal for the long term but also that this approach to creating good health is the best route toward achieving top performance. The program's low-volume, high-intensity training model is based on the following pillars:

- *Developing running skill:* Learn how to reduce the wear and tear of running through the development of good mechanics.
- *Building running endurance without creating injuries:* Avoid injury by avoiding the miles that hurt you rather than help you.
- *Building functional strength, conditioning, and mobility:* By executing varied, functional movements at high intensity, you will build an all-around athletic foundation and state of health that will support faster, healthier running.

- *Focusing on nutrition:* Learn how to feed your body the fuels it needs to enhance health, ensure recovery, and prepare for peak performance.

Who Can Benefit from CFE?

Maybe it is a nagging or debilitating injury that's brought you to this book. Or maybe it is frustration. Perhaps you're not achieving what you'd hoped to accomplish. You've tried other training plans, but they all seemed vaguely similar, and none of them really worked, at least not for long.

Maybe you're curious. You've heard a lot about CrossFit, have friends who swear by it, and wonder if CrossFit Endurance can add something meaningful to your routine.

Or maybe you're a CrossFitter who wants to improve your endurance in order to more effectively run and race.

Whatever brought you here, you're in the right place to learn what CrossFit is all about. In the coming chapters, you'll discover the how and why of CFE, and by the time you reach the end, you'll be ready—should you choose—to become a CFE athlete yourself and to look forward to your next race with the power of CrossFit Endurance behind you. All that is required is that you keep an open mind and a willingness to consider a new approach to your training.

But an open mind does not mean checking your brain at the door. As CFE founder Brian MacKenzie says when challenged on his training philosophy: "Don't take my word for it. Try it out." In other words, be your own scientist and your own experiment.

The contrast between the CFE approach and other training programs disturbs some, but Brian MacKenzie isn't concerned. He's not afraid to shake things up, question accepted conventions, and let the runner decide which approach makes the most sense.

This book will explore the facets of CrossFit Endurance in detail and present basic drills, skills, and methods for getting started with a CFE program. An advantage of CFE's design is that being stronger, having better form, and remaining injury-free naturally increase the chances of running faster, so we'll conclude with several training plans that target specific race distances.

Our intent is not to tell you everything there is to know about these concepts but to provide an overview of the basic mechanics involved in CrossFit Endurance and guidance on how to incorporate them into your own running. Along with these new ideas, we offer some simple experiments so you can test-drive them on your own.

As you make your way through this material, keep in mind that you don't need to adopt every concept and bit of advice presented here. While we do recommend trying out the full CrossFit Endurance program, feel free to incorporate the skill work or strength and conditioning components into your normal schedule to see how they work for you. Doing even a part of this program can lead to improvements in your running, health, and performance.

By the end of this book, we hope that we'll have triggered a more informed conversation about what CrossFit Endurance is all about and how adopting CFE into your program can set you on the path to becoming an unbreakable runner.

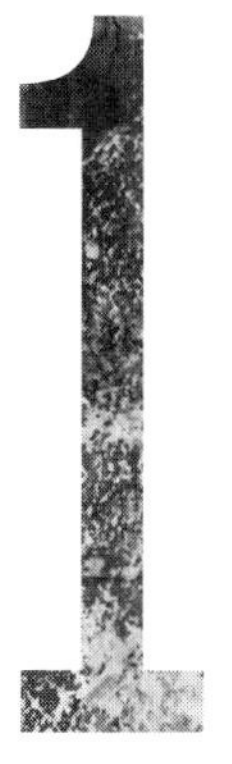

INDESTRUCTIBLE RUNNING FORM

Sure, you can point to great runners who seem to be an anomaly form-wise. But I believe the best runners with the longest careers are those who have the best form. —ALBERTO SALAZAR

In CrossFit Endurance, the idea of approaching running as a skill is more than recommended: It is an essential, high-priority task, emphasized so that a runner both marginalizes the risk of injury and maximizes performance.

Born to Run or Made to Run?

Christopher McDougall opened up a vigorous discussion of form and natural running in his best-selling book, *Born to Run*,[1] in which he describes the legendary ultradistance runners of the Tarahumara tribe who live in Mexico's remote Copper Canyon. Instead of wearing shoes, these runners use homemade footwear crafted from pieces of tire tread. McDougall's description of the Tarahumara and his discussion of the benefits of barefoot running have sparked a debate that continues to rage about what exactly constitutes good running.

Tarahumara runners have been able to run long distances in their ritual events with few apparent ill effects, but, as McDougall reports, they have also competed at the highest level when they've left the Copper Canyon and entered ultramarathons, such as the grueling Leadville Trail 100 Run. For these reasons, barefoot advocates like to point to the Tarahumara as a good example of why all runners should abandon their modern shoes.

However, Daniel Lieberman, an evolutionary biologist at Harvard who is mentioned in McDougall's book, says it's not that simple. When it comes to injury-proof running, Lieberman says, there is no magical fix. "How you run is more important than what is on your feet," he told the *Wall Street Journal* in 2014. "Good running form can happen both ways, you can run poorly barefoot, and extremely well in a shoe."[2]

In other words, the success of the Tarahumara runners is likely due not only to their minimalist shoes but also to other factors, such as their running form, their balanced strength, and the social aspect of their running (similar to that of many African runners).

At the heart of the debate in the competitive running world is whether a runner should mess with running form and mechanics at all. Most coaches have taken the position that it is best to let running form take care of itself. Go out and run a lot, and your form will naturally become more efficient. In this school of thought, we would all become great runners like the Tarahumara if we just ran a lot.

This was precisely the instruction given to my high school track team many years ago. "With every mile you run, you become more efficient," I was told, without further explanation. Like many other young runners, I wasn't told what good form was or how to attain it. I would hear a coach who was watching an admired runner say something like, "What a great stride," but there was no explanation of what makes a stride great.

Ken Doherty, one of the dominant thinkers in track and field technique in the 20th century, set the tone for this hands-off attitude toward form in his *Track and Field Omnibook*: "Running technique is primarily an individual matter. A sound rule of thumb when it comes to running technique is to leave it alone. Do what comes naturally, as long as 'naturally' is mechanically sound."[3]

This position has been challenged, particularly in the last decade. More and more coaches are looking closely at the mechanics of proper running form as the body deals with gravity, balance, and impact force during the running movement. Advocates of this newer approach believe that good runners are made, not born. To obtain proper form and avoid injury, runners should routinely perform movement drills as well as exercises to develop hip and hamstring strength, elasticity in the legs, and range of motion.

Born to run or made to run? Eventually, the argument made its way down to our feet.

How the foot strikes the ground is a central issue among coaches, with the big—arguably overbuilt—running shoes that filled the shelves for decades being a major point of contention. Shoe companies and running magazines have been telling us for years that the antidote to running injury is matching the shape and mechanics of your feet to a specific category of running shoes. Based on the height of your arch and the mobility of your ankles, the formula assures us, you should wear a cushioned neutral shoe, a stability shoe, or a motion control shoe.

However, in an argument detailed at length in McDougall's book, minimalist and barefoot running advocates claim that big shoes allowed runners to land on their heels by cushioning a footfall that otherwise would be too painful to endure. (To test this argument yourself, try landing on your heel while running barefoot and see how far you can go before giving up.)

Landing on the heel is bad because the impact can cause a host of injuries to the ankles, knees, and hips. Even the cushioning afforded by big running shoes can't stave off injury forever. Bit by bit, these cushioned impacts still tear away soft tissue, grinding their way toward injury and possible surgery to repair worn-down cartilage or shredded tendons.

But correcting one's foot strike is not just about reducing impact; it's also about improving running efficiency. Foot strike is a nonissue when mechanics are sound, as the foot lands exactly where it is supposed to—on the ball—without thought. Don't believe me? Jump up and down without thinking about it, as if you were jumping rope, and notice how your feet land.

Think of the line of gravity as it flows downward through your skeleton toward the center of the earth. Now think about your center of gravity as you run, in comparison with where your foot is striking. If you reach out ahead of that line of gravity with each stride—known as "overstriding"—you are hitting the brakes with each step. That's a monumental waste of energy and momentum. Minimal shoes and barefoot running would, according to this school of thought, correct that.

According to this theory, if you shook off your big running shoes and then ran down the street in a barely-there shoe, you'd revert to the natural, barefoot running technique that your ancestors used in their hunter-gatherer days. Rather than reaching out with your leg, jamming your body with a heel strike, and then staying in contact with the ground as you plod your way into the next step, you would instead pop off the ground with quick, light strikes of the forefoot and run for mile after mile without courting injury.

These ideas prompted a sea change in the footwear industry, fueled by pent-up frustration among runners who were spending big money on motion-control running shoes. They kept hoping their new shoes would alleviate their woes but instead ended up disappointed, poorer, and still injured.

The result was the appearance of the "minimalist shoe." Offered with some minor variations by all the major running shoe brands, the minimalist shoe took padding and support to the other extreme, featuring a low or nonexistent heel and less padding in the midsole.

When it comes to claims that a running shoe is a fix for injury problems, some experts are simply skeptical, whether the shoe is minimalistic or not. Dr. Nicholas Romanov (a mentor of Brian MacKenzie) openly scoffed at claims by any manufacturer that a new shoe technology is the solution.

"The human body is made of 100 trillion cells that are the product of millions of years of evolution," Romanov said. "And your pair of $80 shoes that you developed over the last year is going to improve on this?"[4]

In response to such arguments, many coaches and shoe companies have, over the past decade, begun to question the value of a shoe intervention in solving a runner's injury woes. They have pushed the debate by adding in considerations of running form and technique.

It's a complicated topic, and for good reason. The thing is, running is far more complex than it may seem. Consider ASIMO, a humanoid robot designed by Honda to replicate some types of human motion that has given us a peek at the incredible complexity of the "simple" act of running. Jim Gourley, an aeronautical engineer and physicist who has a passion for scouring through peer-reviewed research being done in endurance athletics, is a student of ASIMO. When he considers ASIMO and running form, he does so through the lens of Newtonian physics, analyzing what interferes with momentum and where force is opposed.

"Consider this," Gourley told me, trying to frame the challenges in defining and regulating running form. "You've got some of the most hotshot engineers in the world working on the ASIMO. It takes all of this incredible brain power and advanced science to make a machine that can just walk around and climb some steps. Now, imagine if you decided to put the scientists to the test and make one leg shorter than the other, or compromise the mobility of the robot on one side but not the other. Or throw in some old injury or kink. Those sorts of additional variables could drive them nuts. That's how complicated walking and running is."

Indeed, during one of ASIMO's global demonstrations in 2006, the robot failed to ascend a short flight of steps. Instead, it fell over backward and smashed into the ground. Handlers appeared from the wings with a folding screen to hide the fallen robot.

As the challenges faced by the ASIMO robot illustrate, the movement of running, as simple and everyday as it seems, is incredibly intricate. It's also the third rail of running; bring up running form among a group of runners and coaches and be prepared for a highly

---

Correcting one's foot strike is not just about reducing impact; it's also about improving running efficiency.

---

spirited debate and a lot of strong opinions. Many scientists and coaches are involved in the ongoing discussion, looking not just at what good running form is but at whether or not we should try to tweak it.

Famed Nike coach and USATF 2009 Coach of the Year Alberto Salazar believes in tinkering with form. A former Boston and three-time New York City Marathon champion, Salazar saw his own career flare out while he was still in his 20s. "The way I ran, it wasn't sustainable," Salazar told the *New Yorker* in 2010.[5] "The attitude at the time was: if you were gifted with perfect form, great. If you weren't, you were just kind of stuck." And being kind of stuck, Salazar argued, fast-tracked you toward chronic injury problems. "The knee injury, the hamstring injury—in hindsight, these were the things that killed me."

After retiring as a professional runner, Salazar signed with Nike as head coach of the company's Oregon Project, working to develop a group of potential champion runners, including Dathan Ritzenhein, Kara Goucher, and Galen Rupp. Salazar wasn't sold at first on working on his runners' form, but he noticed something when watching Ethiopian 5K and 10K world record holder and Olympic gold medalist Kenenisa Bekele racing on TV. What caught Salazar's eye was how Bekele's back leg didn't lope upward slowly between strides but had a piston-like action. "While all these other runners had long, trailing legs, his foot was coming right up to his butt," Salazar said. "I thought, is that just coincidence? Or could that perhaps be part of why he's so good?"

Salazar brought in Lance Walker, a Nike expert in sprint mechanics, to work with his distance runners. Walker analyzed Bekele's form and concluded that here was a distance runner—the fastest ever at the 5K distance—who was running like a sprinter.

Walker and Salazar found that the best runners slapped the pavement so quickly and lightly with their forefoot that contact seemed incidental. Walker said it was like a "pogo stick with a stiff spring."

Salazar became a believer in developing good form. In an interview he said, "You show me someone with bad form, and I'll show you someone who's going to have a lot of injuries and a short career."

Salazar pointed to himself as an example. "There has to be one best way of running," he said. "It's got to be like a law of physics. If you deviate too much from that—the way I did in my career—it can be a big handicap. You can be efficient for a while with bad form—maybe with a low shuffle stride—but eventually that's not good for your body. It's going to produce tightness and muscular imbalances and structural problems. Then you get injuries, and if you're not careful—if you don't take care of the muscular and structural issues—the injuries can put you into a downward spiral."

As Salazar began aggressively adjusting and improving the form of his athletes, his runners went on a spree of breakthrough performances, culminating with Galen Rupp's Olympic silver medal in the 10K in London—the first Olympic medal for an American in the 10K in 48 years—and his shattering of the American record for the 10K in May 2014. And who beat Rupp in London? British runner Mo Farah, another of Salazar's form-coached athletes.

The CFE Philosophy: Developing Skill and Technique

But Salazar's experience has not settled the debate about form and whether or not to tinker with it. MacKenzie's thinking on skill as a fix for injury began after years of study under form guru Dr. Nicholas Romanov. MacKenzie's goal wasn't to resolve the debate between the "born" and "made" coaches; he simply wanted to find a better way to train that left his athletes healthier and with fewer injuries.

It didn't take MacKenzie long to figure out what would work best for his athletes; he, too, became a strong proponent of the "made" school of coaching. "Skill is the first thing we teach," says MacKenzie. "If you don't learn the skill first, you have no business running."

The first thing MacKenzie does when coaching a runner through a form overhaul is to eliminate the heel strike. The relevant research has convinced MacKenzie that heel striking is one of the biggest causes of running injuries.

Among the most persuasive research was a 2011 retrospective study in which researchers at Harvard looked at injury rates in competitive distance runners and found an alarming rate of injury: Three out of four of the runners experienced a moderate to severe running injury each year. Particularly revealing was that heel-striking runners accounted for most of the injuries documented by researchers, who wrote, "Those who habitually rear-foot strike had approximately twice the rate of repetitive stress injuries than individuals who habitually forefoot strike."[6]

To avoid these injuries, runners need to aggressively condition the muscles in the core—a topic covered in Chapter 3—and also establish and maintain good posture and running position that replaces a lazy heel strike with a tap-hammer-like running form. This shifts the workload away from smaller muscles such as the calves and hip flexors to large muscles such as the glutes and hamstrings, where it belongs.

To develop proper CFE running technique, MacKenzie's athletes work on mastering the following skills.

Develop a rapid cadence. Ideal running requires a cadence that may be much quicker than you're used to. Shoot for 180 footfalls per minute. Developing the proper cadence will help you achieve more speed because it increases the number of push-offs per minute. It will also help prevent injury, as you avoid overstriding and placing impact force on your heel.

To practice, get an electronic metronome (or download an app for this), set it for 90+ beats per minute, and time the pull of your left foot to the chirp of the metronome.

Develop a proper forward lean. With core muscles slightly engaged to generate a bracing effect, the runner leans forward—from the ankles, not from the waist.

Land underneath your center of gravity. MacKenzie drills his athletes to make contact with the ground as their midfoot or forefoot passes directly under their center of gravity, rather than having their heels strike out in front of the body. When runners become proficient at this, the pounding stops, and the movement of their legs begins to more closely resemble that of a spinning wheel.

Keep contact time brief. "The runner skims over the ground with a slithering motion that does not make the pounding noise heard by the plodder who runs at one speed," the legendary coach Percy Cerutty once said.[7] MacKenzie drills runners to practice a foot pull that spends as little time as possible on the ground. His runners aim to touch down with a light sort of tap that creates little or no sound. The theory is that with less time spent on the ground, the foot has less time to get into the kind of trouble caused by the sheering forces of excessive inward foot rolling, known as "overpronation."

Pull with the hamstring. To create a rapid, piston-like running form, the CFE runner, after the light, quick impact of the foot, pulls the ankle and foot up with the hamstring. Imagine that you had to confine your running stride to the space of a phone booth—you would naturally develop an extremely quick, compact form to gain optimal efficiency. Practice this skill by standing barefoot and raising one leg by sliding your ankle up along the opposite leg. Perform up to 20 repetitions on each leg.

Maintain proper posture and position. Proper posture, MacKenzie says, shifts the impact stress of running from the knees to larger muscles in the trunk, namely, the hips and hamstrings. The runner's head remains up and the eyes focused down the road. With the core muscles engaged, power flows from the larger muscles through to the extremities.

Practice proper position by standing with your body weight balanced on the ball of one foot. Keep the knee of your planted leg slightly bent and your lifted foot relaxed as you hold your ankle directly below your hip. In this position, your body is in proper alignment. Practice holding this position for up to 1 minute on each leg.

Be patient. Choose one day a week for practicing form drills and technique. MacKenzie recommends wearing minimalist shoes to encourage proper form, but not without taking care of the other necessary work. A quick changeover from motion-control shoes to minimalist shoes is a recipe for tendon problems. Instead of making a rapid transition, ease into minimalist shoes by wearing them just one day per week, during skill work. Then slowly integrate them into your training runs as your feet and legs adapt. Your patience will pay off.

But there is more to the story than these guidelines. Developing proper running technique is crucial, but for optimum performance and health, runners need to add one more element: mobility.

Mobility: The New Power Tool for Keeping Runners Healthy

"Are you truly ready for this? Stretching is not important," writes Kelly Starrett, DPT, one of the country's foremost thinkers on the

A RUNNER FOCUSES ON FOOT STRIKE

It was the last week of Brandon Bethke's sophomore year of high school. It was an ordinary sunny day in Orange County, California, and Bethke had a schedule conflict: He had to choose between a soccer game and working out with the running club.

Bethke went to the game. During the game, an opposing player put the full force of a kick into Bethke's ankle. Bethke collapsed to the grass, knowing instantly the ankle was broken, and held the lower bones of his leg together, afraid they were going to shift and fall apart on him.

An ambulance took him away. Surgery was required, and the orthopedic surgeon used two screws to put things back together. Bethke's soccer season was over. He went home in a cast and spent the next 8 weeks healing before he could even think about sports again.

"It was a blessing in disguise," Bethke told me. Two things happened in the course of his remaining time in high school: One, after deciding to let go of soccer for good, he decided to put more effort into running, thinking he might have a shot at the school record in the mile. Two, as he made running his athletic focus, he applied the lessons he had learned from having a severe injury: He would always play offense when it came to building strength and doing whatever was necessary to reduce the chance of an injury. He would also focus on his form.

Says Bethke, when his coach saw that he was heel striking, "he told me to watch the Olympic finals of all the distance races. He asked me how much heel striking was going on."

Bethke embarked on a yearlong journey to overhauling his running form, slowly changing the way he ran so that he was landing on his midfoot, not his forefoot. The change required constant attention to and maintenance of his feet and his calf muscles. To this day, Bethke uses a foam roller, a lacrosse ball, and a massage stick as therapy tools for his running muscles.

As he gradually changed over to striking with the midfoot, he noticed other benefits as well. Not only was he less prone to the chronic ailments that heel striking can cause, but he also unleashed previously untapped speed.

"My speed went through the roof," he says. "My mile dropped from 4:21 to 4:09 to 4:02."

From that point on, for every step of every run, every moment spent lifting weights, every running drill, Bethke focused on how he was moving. "I was in a constant search to improve how the stability muscles fire to make my running better and stronger."

Bethke went on to an All-American collegiate career and to record personal bests of 3:57:34 for the mile and 13:25 for 5000 meters, with his sights set on the marathon and the 2016 Olympics. All with bones held together by screws.

subject of mobility and athletic performance. "Position and the application of position are what matters most. If you can't get into a good position because you're limited or you have a tissue restriction of some kind, stretching alone won't give you the results you want."[8]

In other words, stretching does not effectively target any underlying dysfunction that is the root cause of the chronic injuries that plague runners.

"When I say 'stretching,' I'm referring specifically to end-range static stretching, or hanging out in an end-range static position with zero intention," Starrett writes, meaning that there is no specific purpose involved.

He offers up the typical hamstring stretch as an example: A runner lies on the ground, with hands clasped around one ankle, and draws the leg upward. And then hangs out there. Starrett agrees that this can technically lengthen the hamstring, but holding such an unnatural, "end-range" position doesn't offer the athlete or coach any valuable information about whether or not the runner can get into and sustain a series of good positions while running.

When it comes to the health and performance of a runner, Starrett and MacKenzie broaden the stretching conversation. Rather than focusing just on the length of a muscle such as the hamstring and stretching that muscle after it gets shortened by a workout, they teach runners to think of the big picture. They combine attention to functional strength training with a form of self-performed physical therapy that in recent years has become known as "mobility."

Mobility practice involves improving range of motion and establishing new, ideal motor patterns. It does this by overcoming the restrictions and problems—like tight hips or compromised ankle range of motion—that may prevent good body position. Pursuing these targets may include changing daily habits, requiring that closer attention be paid to nonrunning movements and positions throughout the day, such as how you stand, walk, and sit.

Think of a runner's legs as pogo sticks, says physicist Gourley. With the essentials of a CFE running technique in mind—a faster stride rate, less up-and-down motion, and a snappy foot pull—the runner aims to bounce along as efficiently as possible. This pogo stick–like bounce is elasticity.

For runners who are habitual heel strikers, elasticity forces of the lower legs are largely dormant. Rather than popping off the ground, a heel strike involves longer contact with the ground in the form of a land-to-rolling push-off. It's a lazy way to run.

As discussed earlier, the wearing of bulky running shoes does not help; often overbuilt in the heel, these shoes enable heel striking because they shield runners from the pain that would otherwise naturally ensue when the heel hits the ground. Over time, being a heel striker allows for a degree of atrophy in the "coils" of Gourley's pogo-stick model.

For runners growing up in Kenya's Rift Valley, running barefoot 6 miles back and forth to school every day on dirt, elasticity is well taken care of. The coils would be charged and ready. But for runners clunking around in motion-control shoes for a significant period of time, elasticity can wither away.

Explaining this concept, physical therapist Jay Dicharry says in his book, "Poor control of the position of your spine and hips means you can't take advantage of the storage and release of elastic energy that enable you to run efficiently."[9]

But poor posture is responsible for all sorts of running problems, Dicharry says. For example, poor posture causes the center of gravity to shift backward, encouraging overstriding and the resulting heel strike and increase in injury risk. "It impairs your ability to activate the muscles that stabilize the spine and the lower legs," says Dicharry, "by as much as 50 percent."

From his lab in Bend, Oregon, Dicharry studies each athlete he works with from the ground up, looking for imbalances and weaknesses that are allowing good performance to leak out. Strength and conditioning are a big part of good performance, but Dicharry maintains that core strength work isn't much help unless you are using good positions in your running. Says Dicharry, "Better posture *means* better muscle recruitment."

Over the past decade, voices like Dicharry's have opened up a new discussion regarding the power of mobility—in the feet, legs, and hips. To restore mobility and elasticity, they say, runners need to spend time massaging their feet, calf muscles, hamstrings, quads, and hips, and then do exercises to develop and sustain good positions with the hips and lower spine.

A mobility program, like the one outlined here within the CFE model, trains good muscle recruitment patterns through functional strength exercises to make better use of the springlike elasticity that we can tap from our legs.

Minimalist shoes can also make a contribution to mobility. While traditional shoes provide considerable control over foot movement, minimalist shoes have multidirectional flexibility that is designed to let the foot move as naturally as possible. Ultimately, this leads to greater mobility.

But isn't a running shoe supposed to correct for runners' biomechanical shortcomings? That's been the idea, but as Chris McDougall reported in *Born to Run*, there is no research to support the belief that motion-control shoes and stability shoes do anything of the sort.

In fact, the U.S. Army Public Health Command has conducted three studies, involving 9,000 trainees in the air force, the army, and the marines, to see if matching up a recruit's foot with a prescribed shoe made any difference. The conclusion? Dr. Bruce Jones, a runner and the manager of the U.S. Army's Injury Prevention Program, said the results were black and white: The motion-control/stability shoe framework for runners had no basis in reality.[10] "It turned out to be a sports myth," Jones told the Army News Service.

The new thinking, incorporated in the design of the Nike Free running shoe—a so-called barefootlike shoe—is that the only way to correct for biomechanical weaknesses is to revive the natural strength and mobility of the foot. Motion-control shoes and orthotics may provide some temporary relief, this line of thinking goes, but they won't solve the problem over the long term.

This stance is thoroughly embraced by MacKenzie. The key, he says, is patience. If you've been running in a stiff stability shoe with a raised heel, and maybe even with an orthotic, you can't just jump into a pair of Nike Frees or flat-soled Inov-8s. Rather, a runner needs to introduce a minimalist shoe in small doses, allowing the foot to slowly adapt over time by rekindling ankle flexibility and arch strength. Mobility exercises can help support this process.

So for a runner pursuing maximum performance, recovery, and injury prevention, stretching alone just doesn't cut it. The road to better running involves adopting a more complete program.

A Start-up Guide for a Basic Mobility Routine for Runners

Doing mobility therapy is not glamorous, and it probably won't leave you with a runner's high. It's work, and for some it can be quite dull. But if you consistently do these movements three times a week or more, you will begin to see improvement over time, and you won't have your running interrupted by an injury time-out. In the long run, that will make it all worthwhile.

To complete this routine, you will need a foam roller, a massage stick, and a lacrosse ball or massage ball.

- Use your watch or your smart phone to set a timer to beep every minute. This will be your taskmaster as you work your way through these movements.

- Roll the ball under each foot for 1 minute. Hunt out any hot spots and apply pressure to those spots.

- Using the massage stick, go after the calf muscles, 1 minute per leg. If you find any deep knots, spend extra time rolling deeply across the knot with the massage ball or lacrosse ball.
- Lie facedown on the floor, with your thighs resting on the foam roller. Roll out your quadriceps muscles, spending 1 minute on each side.
- Use the foam roller to roll out your iliotibial (IT) bands, which extend from the hip to the knee on the outside of the leg. Spend 1 minute on each leg.
- Use the roller to roll out the hamstrings, 1 minute per side.
- Spend a final couple of minutes rolling out each hip and also the lower back. A softball or softball-sized mobility ball is another tool that can be used to work out any knots in the gluteus muscles.

Improving mobility involves more than just doing these movements, however; it's also about making a few subtle but important lifestyle changes.

First of all, whenever possible, go barefoot. When you're at home, walk around with no shoes (if you wish to wear socks, use toe socks so your toes can move freely). If you have a habit of standing or walking with your feet like a duck (external rotation) or a pigeon (internal rotation), work to correct your stance, standing and walking with your feet in a neutral position.

Learn to engage your core muscles. MacKenzie recommends turning on the muscles supporting your trunk to about a constant 25 percent level of engagement. Do this by squeezing the glute muscles and locking the ab muscles, as if you were bracing for a punch to the stomach, then dial it down to about a quarter effort. This simple sequence will brace the pelvis into healthy position. Do this when you're standing, when you are walking or running, and before you sit down with a well-braced lower spine. This will help you stabilize the spine and keep your extremities—including your feet—in the proper position.

HOW TO TRANSITION INTO A MINIMALIST SHOE

In the aftermath of *Born to Run*'s success, droves of runners who had been tethered to stability shoes with raised heels went a little crazy, thinking they could instantly toss their Asics Gel Kayanos and slip on a pair of featherweight "zero-drop" shoes, and their feet would be revitalized.

Since then, a good deal of mainstream criticism has been leveled at minimalist running shoes. But as Dr. Nick Campitelli—a long-distance runner and podiatrist in Akron, Ohio—cautions, this is a recipe for disaster. In an interview, Campitelli, the author of an e-book titled *Running in a Minimalist Shoe,* offered the following suggestions to those wanting to make the jump.

Campitelli says to use the 10 percent rule: Transition into flat (aka zero-drop) shoes with incremental changes that take place at the rate of no more than 10 percent per week. For example, if you run 4 miles per day, 6 days a week, you would start off each run in a pair of zero-drop shoes, running .4 miles. After that, you'd switch to the shoes you've been using and complete the run. After a week, you would spend an additional 10 percent of the run in the minimalist shoes.

Dr. Campitelli suggests that the process should take at least 6 to 8 weeks, and an even less aggressive time line may be prudent. It's all about how your body responds to the new set of demands being placed upon it.

Minimize sitting, even though this can be a significant challenge, given our modern workplace. Extended amounts of sitting can reduce flexibility and strength in the hamstrings and hip flexors, which cascades into a multitude of weaknesses and problems.

Do your best to counteract this situation by getting out of your office chair periodically to do a quick mobility exercise. Also, take a lacrosse ball to the office or on long plane flights and spend time jamming it into the hamstring or sweet spot of a hip while you're sitting.

GO BACK TO GO FORWARD

Give some thought to a game or sport from your childhood that involved less specificity and more all-around athleticism than running. Did you ride a skateboard, love climbing, or play basketball? Were you a gymnast? Returning to these sports in some fashion can be more than nostalgic; it can lead to being a better runner and a better athlete in general.

With a traditional running program built solely on distance running, playing other sports can lead to injury because although you may be a fit runner, you may lack the kind of strength and fitness that other sports require. However, laying a foundation with CFE helps you restore certain dimensions of athleticism that you may not have enjoyed since childhood. Because CFE includes strength training, power training, gymnastics training, and more, it provides an opportunity to complement your running with a different type of sport. And, in turn, participating in those sports can train your body to once again move strongly in multiple planes.

Competing in the sports of your youth once again might not only be great fun; it can give an intangible boost to your running performance.

To help reduce your sitting time, consider buying a standing desk. Ultrarunning star Dean Karnazes owns one. "I rarely sit," he says. He uses the standing desk for e-mail, managing his business, and writing. He breaks up his workday with blasts of functional movement exercises.

MacKenzie practices the same sort of doctrine. "I never sit. If I'm relaxing on the couch at the end of the day watching TV, I'm lying down, not sitting."

In this chapter, we've built the foundation for the run workouts that will follow. In the next chapter, we'll begin describing those workouts and how CrossFit Endurance differs from many "traditional" running programs.

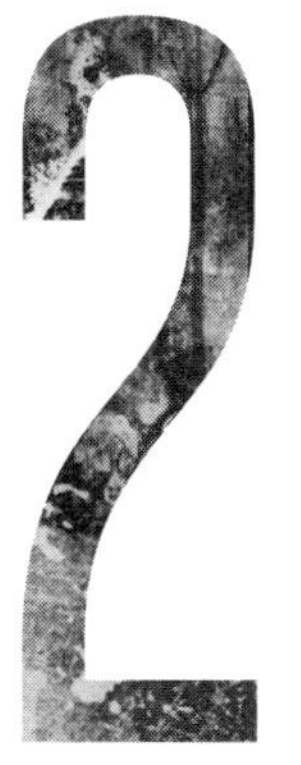

ENDURANCE WITH TEETH

Somebody once asked me to write an article about overtraining. That's the easiest article I've ever written. It's two words: Avoid it.

—DR. JACK DANIELS, FAMED RUNNING COACH AND EXERCISE PHYSIOLOGIST

CrossFit Endurance is not just a program that builds strength and mobility. It is also a running program, although one that is likely to seem unusual to most runners. In CFE, mileage is relatively low, but every run is targeted to deliver maximum endurance and speed benefits.

Traditional Training as a Risky Business

To run long distance well, you need to stimulate changes in the muscle cells, the heart, the blood, and the joints and bones. To achieve this result, most running programs, from those prescribed for beginners and first-time marathoners to those for seasoned, advanced runners, are built around a core of easy to medium-paced running, with an emphasis on progressively building up the weekly mileage total.

As we discussed in the introduction, this approach is known as long, slow distance (LSD) running.

The defining characteristic of LSD running is that it is aerobic, which means that the exercise is so low in intensity that the oxidative energy system—that is, the low-gear, fuel-burning process that works only in the presence of oxygen—can handle the demand over an extended period. This is considered crucial for endurance athletes because the fuel used by the body in the oxidative energy system is stored carbohydrate and fat—sources that are usually plentiful. If you can train your body to utilize a higher percentage of fat, you're much more likely to avoid bonking during your long races, and that improves your chance of crossing the finish line. A principle value of LSD running is that it increases the body's fat-burning efficiency.

An often-recommended method of ensuring that a run is in the LSD zone is the talk test: If you can comfortably carry on a conversation while out for a 1-hour run, then you are keeping the run aerobic. If you can't handle conversing because the intensity is too high, the run is too intense and has become anaerobic.

As the term implies, anaerobic workouts rely on fuels that can be burned without the presence of oxygen, such as blood sugar. These are high-octane fuels, but they run out quickly, and the body needs time to fully replenish them. For these reasons, they are not the fuel of choice for endurance athletes.

To get a feel for what an anaerobic workout is like, try sprinting at your top speed for as long as you can. After a minute or so, you'll be gasping for air and feeling burning in your legs and lungs. There's no keeping up such maximum intensity for long.

In the traditional model of endurance training, a heavy load of LSD running is recommended to prepare the body for speed work and eventually racing. This approach supposedly relies on the principle of specificity, discussed in the introduction. This principle, which exists within the greater bedrock of sports medicine and sports training theory, basically states that to improve in an activity, you need to devote the bulk of your training time to that activity.

For this reason, running coaches have long pointed to crosstraining as a sensible alternative to maintain fitness while injured but not as a good substitute for running itself. According to tradition, to get better at running, you have to run, and the more the better. Many elite marathoners take this advice to extremes, logging as much as 100 to 150 miles per week.

Coaches who focus on LSD say that their training programs are best for training long-distance runners because LSD improves a runner's ability to stay in the aerobic zone and to burn carbohydrate and fat most efficiently. They claim that LSD runs deliver these positive adaptations:

- *Improved oxygen intake:* This is measured by how much oxygen you need to sustain a certain pace, known by its scientific designation, VO_2max.

- *Changes in the skeletal muscle cells:* This occurs chiefly as "mitochondrial biogenesis," which is the process by which the body packs more mitochondria into each muscle cell. This is important to runners because the mitochondria, nicknamed "the powerhouse of the cell" in innumerable biology textbooks, are where fuel is converted to energy. Simply put, the more mitochondria you have in a cell, the more energy that cell has available to produce work.

- *Increased bone density:* Bones are living tissue and respond to reasonable amounts of stress by increasing their density.

More running means more stimuli to the bones to increase their density.

- *Improved tendon and ligament strength:* Tendons attach muscles to bone, and ligaments hold bones together—all with the important aim of handling the impact stress of running. These, too, adapt positively to increased running by becoming denser and more durable.
- *Increased density of the capillary network:* Improving this network will increase the body's ability to rush oxygen-rich blood to the running muscles, an obvious advantage for long-distance runners.
- *Maximal fat burning:* A highly desired adaptation claimed to result from LSD training is an uptick in the metabolism of stored fat. This appeals to novice runners for health and appearance reasons. For advanced long-distance runners, an increased ability to utilize stored fat means having access to an almost inexhaustible supply of energy.

Undeniably, LSD running produces a training effect. Generally speaking, lots of LSD running over periods of weeks and months—LSD being defined here as 50 to 60 miles per week and up—can produce the above-mentioned adaptations as long as injury or the precursors to injury don't creep in. But that is a major caveat. As we discussed in Chapter 1, even otherwise healthy runners who ignore form and strength work leave themselves open to eventually developing problems. Nevertheless, an LSD program works for some runners, at least for a while. Then, for many of them, the toll of high-mileage running kicks in, and they join the ranks of those many other runners for whom an LSD plan is a road to ruin. That's because along with its benefits, high-mileage running brings an increased risk of injury.

My own experience with high-mileage training, which I related in the Writer's Note, from initial running success to eventual physical breakdown, is, unfortunately, an all-too-common one among long-distance runners.

For marathoners in particular, the news only gets worse. A 2007 study published in *Sports Medicine* found that 90 percent of marathoners had incurred an injury while training for a race.[1] Most common among their ailments are injuries to the knees (25 to 35 percent), the calves and shins (20 percent), the IT bands (10 percent), and the feet and arches (10 percent).[2]

Why does this happen? Because high-mileage running can reduce an athlete's mobility, range of motion, and explosive power, resulting in muscular imbalances and postural weaknesses. These, in turn, lead to injury, especially when the runner isn't also working on form, strength, and mobility.

But that's not all. High-mileage training can have negative effects on overall health. It can increase stress on the endocrine system, accelerate aging, and compromise the immune system.

Finally, an all-too-common conclusion to this story is that even if runners manage to avoid injury while training under an LSD program, they may yet be disappointed on race day as they fail to run to their potential. That's because after the initial benefits of cardiovascular improvement are realized, the only kind of strength that easy base running develops is strength for slow speeds.

Not surprisingly, many coaches and runners have been looking for an alternative to the LSD model.

Finding Another Way

An emerging body of evidence indicates that there is indeed another way to get favorable results from training, and even improve speed, without risking overuse injury. The key is to let go of the addiction to LSD and begin to envision a new way of building endurance.

A close reading of the emerging data shows that runners, both amateur and elite, are able to cultivate better race performance, reduce injury, and lengthen their running careers by taking a low-mileage, high-intensity approach to their training that uses strength to boost coordination, speed, and running economy. Over and over again, solid scientific research has revealed that higher-quality training can achieve the same positive results as LSD training, but with a lower incidence of injury.

Here's how high-intensity training matches up to some of the claims of the LSD method.

Increasing bone density. While proponents of LSD running claim improved bone health as a result of their training method, LSD running can also result in the opposite: a stress fracture caused by an excessive training load.

Power training, in contrast, does a better job of increasing bone density without causing injury. Studies performed at the University

---

Rather than a 100 percent peak once or twice a year, the CFE runner remains at 95 percent of working potential and can race year-round.

---

of Michigan's Bone and Joint Injury Prevention and Rehabilitation Center revealed that training programs that include gymnastics, weight training, and jumping and bounding exercises—known as "plyometric" training—improve bone-density profiles.[3] These are exactly the types of training modes that CFE prescribes.

Further, because these exercises don't involve the level of repetition that hours of running require, the high-intensity/power method is less likely to cause stress fractures.

Building tendon and ligament strength. LSD running may help strengthen these structures, but as exercise physiologist Tudor Bompa has pointed out, 6 weeks of weight training can also generate substantial connective tissue gains.[4] Further, because a weight training and plyometrics progression can target and improve specific tendons and ligaments, a CFE-type program may be more efficient and effective at improving these structures than just pounding the sidewalk for as many miles as you can.

Improving capillary growth. While the traditional base-training model asserts that a benefit of LSD training is the increase of blood-delivering capillaries surrounding running muscles, researchers have demonstrated that high-intensity exercise can increase capillary networks within 4 weeks around both fast-twitch and slow-twitch muscle fibers.[5]

Maximizing fat burning. A 1994 study by the Physical Activities Science Laboratory in Quebec revealed the fat-burning power of interval training, in which high-intensity training periods are alternated with short rest periods.[6]

In the study, one group of subjects executed a 20-week program of endurance training workouts at medium intensity. Another group performed 15 weeks of high-intensity interval training workouts. The subjects in the second group burned off fat at nine times the rate of the low-intensity group. This study effectively undermined the notion that the "fat-burning" zone is restricted to the realm of low-intensity exercise at a heart rate of 120 beats per minute and that LSD training is the only way to effectively achieve this result. In other words, if your goal is to train your body to burn fat, LSD isn't the only, or even the best, way to go about doing it.

Improving running economy. Researchers Véronique Billat and Jean-Pierre Koralsztein have shown that slow- to moderate-paced running is inferior to fast-paced workouts in producing greater levels of economy.

By fast-paced, Billat and Koralsztein mean training at 95 to 100 percent of your VO_2max—a very intense effort. "VO_2max sessions do not work on a single variable," they explain, "but rather improve several key physiological variables in concert: VO_2max, running economy, and lactate-threshold speed were all upgraded through the use of a single (that is, more intense) running pace."[7]

In sum, for many of the claims staked out by LSD, high-intensity training offers an alternate route toward producing the same basic adaptions, with less of the incessant pounding that leads to injury.

Trading in Miles for Intensity

For a low-volume program to be effective, however, it can't be easy. Although less time is required, that time will be spent doing challenging, exhausting work. But research shows that this kind of high-intensity training has teeth.

A 2005 study conducted by Kirsten Burgomaster is one of the central reports to support this principle.[8] In Burgomaster's study, mitochondrial growth—that is, an increase in the body's ability to produce energy on the cellular level—was measured by the amount of the enzyme citrate synthase that was found in muscle samples from a group of subjects exposed to 2 weeks of sprint interval training.

The subjects performed just 6 workouts over the period, with each workout consisting of 2 to 4 minutes of very intense sprints. The results? A 38 percent increase in just 14 days.

In simple terms, these athletes had achieved dramatically higher energy levels during muscular work in just a few weeks of training. As Ed Coyle, of the University of Texas, remarked in a review of the research,[9] this was a breakthrough insight into the big-picture aerobic effect of anaerobic work.

Another study, conducted by Leena Paavolainen and Heikki Rusko at the Finnish Research Institute for Olympic Sports, linked 9 weeks of explosive training with an 8 percent gain in economy at a 5K running pace, the largest gain ever described in published research.[10]

What drives these kinds of gains? Owen Anderson, author of *Running Science* and elite coach to several Kenyan runners, offers an explanation. The emphasis on a high-volume base, he writes, represents "old-school thinking with the focus of training centered almost entirely on cardiovascular and oxygen-usage development and almost no emphasis placed on neuromuscular progress,"[11] which is the ability of the runner to recruit leg muscles in a way that boosts power, coordination, and speed. Fast running and explosive power training spur this type of improvement.

The neuromuscular progress noted in Paavolainen and Rusko's research has also contributed to our growing understanding of fatigue. One of the reasons marathoners have been encouraged to run as many miles as they can during training is due to the notion that it will build strength that can make them impervious to muscle breakdown in long runs and races. But new thinking is challenging this assumption.

The central question being asked is why a marathoner tends to hit the wall during a race. Hitting the wall, or bonking, is when, somewhere around mile 20 in the race, a runner feels unable to maintain his or her pace, or even to continue at all.

Many coaches who advocate LSD training believe the fault lies in the runner's failure to log enough miles in training. However, research indicates that fewer than 20 percent of motor units are recruited in a marathoner's legs at any time during competition, so it's not a matter of the runner having failed to build an endurance base. Instead, exercise physiologists now hypothesize that the source of the problem is the failure of the runner to more fully engage these neural connections during training.

According to a new theory that's attracting a lot of attention among researchers, such as Tim Noakes,[12] the way to reach a higher level of performance is not just to pile on more miles but instead to focus on stimulating something called the "neural governor." This is the region of the brain that is believed to be responsible for calibrating exercise intensity and neural output.

This governor is a kind of gatekeeper for physical exertion. When training or racing gets too intense, the neural governor generates feelings of fatigue to slow things down. To get faster or run farther, a runner must overcome the limits set by the neural governor. This is not an unrealistic goal. As suggested in a research review in 2008, the neural governor can be trained to allow you to dish out more energy with less fatigue.[13]

What this boils down to is that endurance athletes hoping to achieve optimal levels of performance can no longer focus only on their hearts and muscles; they must also advance neural output to its highest level. Research on optimizing neural output is limited, but it is known that high-intensity, explosive strength training—the kind found in CFE workouts—upgrades neural output more than other forms of strengthening.

What About Periodization?

According to the classic marathon training model, LSD runs are part of the overall organization of the training cycle, usually lasting 6 months or longer and partitioned into three or four phases. Each phase targets a specific energy system or athletic component of running.

The first phase consists of several months of easy to medium-effort aerobic "base" running such as we've been discussing. This is followed by a phase of hill or strength work, followed by anaerobic speed and a peaking phase, which in theory would be when a runner would reach his or her maximum point of development, ideally on race day. After the race, the cycle returns to easy jogging and a new phase one.

In CFE, however, rather than long buildups to one or two peaks per year, the runner trains according to a weekly template that incorporates all of the target components of training. All of the physiological ingredients of running and the different energy systems, including anaerobic and aerobic energy pathways, are worked across a 1- or 2-week period to maintain a constant upward trajectory. Rather than a 100 percent peak once or twice a year, the CFE runner remains at 95 percent of working potential and can race year-round.

The Bottom Line

Research has been making an increasingly strong case for the proposition that when it comes to long-distance training, fewer miles can lead to better running, as long as intensity is boosted.

In building a training program that uses less to get more, we can find an appropriate guiding principle in an idea taken from the medical world: the minimum effective dose. This pharmaceutical guideline emphasizes taking the smallest dose that will produce the desired outcome. This concept is also central to CFE.

A key benefit of adhering to this policy as a runner—making every step count—is a reduced risk of injury. We've discussed how statistics show that being a distance runner introduces the risk of getting hurt. In searching for a program that will deliver results, abiding by the minimum-effective-dose principle suggests spending your running miles and overall training time getting the absolute most bang for your buck.

Be thrifty—stingy, even—and parcel out your training schedule in a way that yields the most performance improvement with the smallest dose.

As you'll see in the programs that follow later in this book, this is a guiding principle of CFE training.

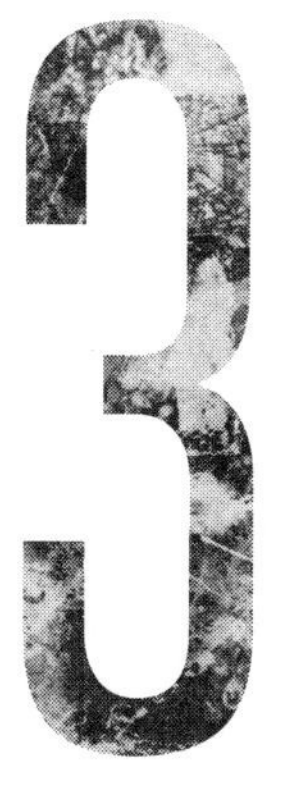

STRENGTH & CONDITIONING WORKOUTS FOR THE CFE RUNNER

No scientific study has ever linked advances in running-training volume beyond 57 miles per week with increases in running performance-related physiological variables, yet elite and serious runners routinely climb the so-called volume ladder beyond this point instead of focusing on tweaking the intensity of their training and developing an outstanding run-specific strength program.

—OWEN ANDERSON, *RUNNING SCIENCE*

In the CrossFit Endurance program, strength and conditioning workouts replace most of the low-intensity aerobic running that appears in conventional training plans. Rather than relying on sheer mileage to produce adaptations that allow a runner to run longer and faster, the CFE runner does short, high-intensity interval workouts using functional[1] strength training to produce similar circulatory, muscular, and respiratory adaptions without all of the pounding.

For a more effective base period in your run training, one in which you build economy, strength, endurance, and resistance to injury, dump excessive slow running and take up circuit strength training.

Circuit training advances aerobic capacity, lactate threshold, running economy, and VO_2max and also improves coordination—making for a faster stride rate and better running form—and neuromuscular development. And all this can be accomplished with less pounding of the pavement and the potential injuries that come with that.

Based on the anecdotal lore of running and information gleaned from research, there is one thing we know for sure about running lots of miles per week: The more you run, the more likely you are to get injured.[2]

This is a vexing problem for a runner motivated to improve performance. Let's say a runner wants to break 3 hours for the marathon, or 40 minutes for the 10K. For decades, he or she has been told that in order to run faster, the mileage must go up. There's a "live by the sword, die by the sword" bargain involved in that, however. With more miles comes a greater risk of injury.

Consider one runner's log, a four-year stretch dating back to 2009. In it are chronicled two strained hip flexors, a strained right Achilles tendon, Achilles surgery, a strained calf, a broken third metatarsal, a strained left Achilles tendon, nerve damage in the left ankle, a "tweaked" hamstring, and sciatic nerve pain.

These injuries do not belong to an uninformed, overly ambitious newcomer but to American distance star Amy Yoder Begley, a 2008 Olympian. Despite being a full-time professional, with access to the best sports medicine, massage, and coaching that a Nike sponsorship could provide, Begley, who seemed born to run, found herself crossing a never-ending minefield of problems.

In 2013, journalist Phil Latter commented on Begley's injuries, arguing that we need to abandon the common thinking when it comes to running and health. "There isn't a fine line between health and injury: there is no line," he wrote.[3] "We are all, at all times, on a continuum between being unable to walk to running freely without pain—the closest we can come to being 'injury-free'—yet even then we're managing defects, weaknesses, imbalances, scar tissue and the stresses of the activity itself."

For the determined age-group runner, out to raise mileage to increase performance, who has a career and a family and numerous concomitant demands on his or her time, the Begley story (which is similar to the injury-ridden tales of other current elite runners, such as Ryan Hall and Dathan Ritzenhein) raises a compelling question: If a pro with all the professional support imaginable can't evade chronic injury, what hope does an average runner have?

The frequently offered injury prevention buffer of a 10-minute core strength routine and a brand-new pair of shoes just doesn't sell. This very problem led Brian MacKenzie to ask: Is there a more efficient training path to elicit the desired adaptations of endurance and strength that doesn't beat the hell out of your body?

Integrating CrossFit

MacKenzie's initial foray into the world of ultrarunning was a traditional one from a training point of view: heavy mileage and zero time spent in a weight room. MacKenzie loved being on the trails for extensive periods, and he found a deep satisfaction in the spiritual exploration that racing for 12 hours and longer can offer. What started to drive him crazy, though, was how messed up a race left him.

He could finish a 50K, a 50-miler, a 100-miler, or an Ironman triathlon, but after the race he was physically destroyed, flat on the sofa for a week and limping when he had to walk. He also registered huge amounts of muscle loss, strength loss, and the destruction of his flexibility.

If training at high mileage was supposed to deliver a foundation of strength, why was he so broken? Dipping into his former athletic life as a power lifter, MacKenzie began to experiment, adding deadlifts and heavy-barbell squats into his training. He threw himself into the study of running technique, seeking to minimize, through proper form, the wear and tear that resulted from pounding the pavement.

MacKenzie dumped his high-carbohydrate diet and played with diets that helped reduce the body's inflammation levels rather than jack them up. He used all the technologies he could get his hands on, from heart rate monitors to pulse oximeters, high-altitude tents, metabolic testing, and blood lactate analyzers. MacKenzie also began testing out different models of run training. One of his running experiments included a series of 20-second all-out intervals on a treadmill cranked to a grade of 8 percent or higher, adhering to what is called the Tabata protocol, a relentless series of 20-second sprints with mere 10-second rests, which blasted blood lactate levels to extremely high levels with the intent of improving VO_2max.

Circuit training advances aerobic capacity, lactate threshold, running economy, and VO_2max and also improves coordination and neuromuscular development.

MacKenzie started seeing results, both in his own running and in his coaching. His logs showed a massive difference that weight training made in his body's ability to absorb the punishment of running. His recovery times quickened, and annoying pains vanished.

But what really distinguished this program from all the other training schedules that MacKenzie found was his inclusion of CrossFit workouts. “It was the missing piece,” he says. CrossFit merged weight training, body-weight gymnastics movements, and cardio intervals into high-speed circuit workouts. He found he could afford to make huge cuts in his mileage levels, allowing the CrossFit to help develop and sustain his endurance. The power lifting and Olympic lifting, MacKenzie discovered, produced a physical durability that far surpassed what long training runs had given him. Through the new musculoskeletal sturdiness that came with heavy overhead squats and deadlifts, he held good running form longer in races and recovered quickly. He could run a 100K or longer and not feel destroyed for days on end.

In MacKenzie’s early version of what would later be termed CrossFit Endurance, strength work was not an ancillary component. It mixed conditioning into the strength piece and made it central.

Rather than build a base with long, slow miles and fill a week of training with as much running as possible to pump up weekly mileage, MacKenzie relied on CrossFit for a broadband training stimulus. The running portion was stripped down to two or three speed-endurance-style workouts per week: a tempo/time trial run and two interval workouts.

Low-mileage/high-quality running programs have been around in one form or another for many years. In the past 20 years, cross-training has been commonly used to make up the difference when a runner (often the injury-plagued runner) looks for a way to reduce mileage without sacrificing fitness. In this brand of low-mileage training, the runner replaces easy runs (sometimes referred to as “junk runs” because of their low quality and intensity) with cycling, swimming, cross-country skiing, or even in-line skating. The intensity is the same—the workouts are meant to simulate the aerobic effort of easy runs but to provide relief from the pounding.

MacKenzie's model differs in that CrossFit workouts impact the aerobic and anaerobic energy systems, not just the aerobic. They also stress the runner with an ongoing variety of functional movement patterns that improve speed, coordination, and power by pulling, pushing, jumping, running, lifting, and throwing. These compound movements recruit muscles throughout the body in new and complex patterns.

Unlike running, which involves movement on a single plane as the arms and legs move forward and back, CrossFit involves lateral and rotational movements. The result is new strength in areas that used to be weak and a reduced risk of the types of injuries to knees and hips that can result from poor lateral strength. Per MacKenzie's philosophy—and his own experiences—this use of CrossFit spurs endurance improvements even in runners doing less mileage.

What started quietly began to grow as, over time, many people began to see the wisdom of MacKenzie's approach. By 2014, MacKenzie's CrossFit Endurance method was guiding 120 training teams around the world, with an additional 35,000 to 40,000 athletes following the program via the CFE web site and social media.

Wait, Weights?

If one had to choose a single adjective to describe the quintessential long-distance runner, what word might that be? "Skinny" would be a good option. Although there are exceptions, when you look at an elite field of long-distance runners—marathoners for sure—you see some very skinny people. Some might use weights, but many never

THE INNOVATORS

The athlete who uses the zombie-like method lacks all the creativity and spontaneity that he was gifted with as a child.

—Larry Myers, describing Australian coaching great Percy Cerutty's view on one-dimensional run training

The breakthrough moment for Brian MacKenzie in developing the CrossFit Endurance method was to look at running and racing with fresh eyes and with a willingness to examine what may work and what does not, regardless of what the common practice has been.

While much of Brian's thinking is fresh, he is not the first coach to apply this approach to running; over the past century, other innovators have also challenged the established orthodoxy. Although they came from a variety of backgrounds—a civil servant, a factory worker, a shoe cobbler, a high school biology teacher, an engineer—they showed that creative experimentation can produce results.

PERCY CERUTTY was born in 1895 in a suburb of Melbourne, Australia. When he was 6 years old, he contracted double pneumonia, which left him with excruciating pain in his left lung when he tried to run. After failing an army physical during World War I, he worked as a civil servant. In his early 40s, Cerutty began to lose weight, suffer severe energy loss, and battle migraine headaches. Doctors thought he might be dying. Cerutty changed his diet and started running. He sprinted up sand dunes and performed gymnastics routines. In his 50s, he started coaching others with his program. One of his athletes, Herb Elliott, won gold in the 1960 Olympic 1500 meters and set a world record. Cerutty himself ran a 5:32 mile—at age 62.

Cerutty believed that a major weakness for many distance runners was lack of upper-body strength as well as a lack of focus on quality running. Runners in Cerutty's program were directed to do

CONTINUED

CONTINUED

intense weight lifting twice a week, perform gymnastics, and run at different paces.

EMIL ZÁTOPEK was born in 1922 in Czechoslovakia. By age 16, he was done with school and working in a shoe factory. When he was chosen to run a 1-mile factory race, he surprised himself by coming in second, and he caught the running bug.

He joined a local athletics club but worked up his own style of training consisting almost exclusively of high-rep interval work, such as doing 60 repeats of 400 meters with brief recoveries. Other Zátopek training secrets were running in army boots and, when the weather was awful, piling towels into a bathtub and running in place in the tub.

In the 1948 Olympic Games, Zátopek won the gold medal in the 10,000 meters and the silver medal in the 5000 meters. In the 1952 Games, he won gold in the 5000 and 10,000 and then, on a lark, hopped into the marathon. He won the gold in 2:23. He remains the only runner to sweep those three events at the same Olympics.

PETER COE was an engineer in Sheffield, England. He wasn't a runner, but his son Sebastian was. When Seb was 12, he started running with a local club that had him doing lots of high-mileage running. Peter didn't like what he saw. He pulled his son from the program and started experimenting. He developed a training program that emphasized high-quality running over volume. There were no 100-mile training weeks; rather, Seb's training rarely exceeded 50 miles per week. It focused on speed-endurance training—fast runs and fast interval training. It also included circuit training in the gym, including burpees, plyometrics, and weight training.

Sebastian Coe raced in distances from the 400 meter to the 3K and went on to set 13 world records and win 4 Olympic medals, including gold in the 1500 meters in both 1980 and 1984.

Peter Coe's method included high-intensity functional strength training in a circuit—a precursor to MacKenzie's CFE approach. Coe believed that the benefits of circuit training included better posture, improved endurance and muscle recruitment, better coordination, and stronger connective tissues. A Peter Coe–designed circuit workout consisted of 2 to 5 circuits of exercises such as dips, back extensions, sit-ups, push-ups, squat thrusts, burpees, and a rope climb.

BILL BOWERMAN studied journalism and played football in college. After serving as an officer in World War II, he took a job in 1948 coaching the University of Oregon track team. Over the next 24 years, he produced 33 Olympians and 16 athletes who ran sub-4-minute miles. Among his many innovations was the development of the hard/easy approach to training, in which athletes vary the intensity of their training in scheduled cycles.

Bowerman also tinkered with sports drinks, lightweight apparel, and running shoes. He partnered with one of his former runners to market his running shoes in a company that eventually came to be called Nike.

touch a barbell, and they surely look it. This is one reason the emphasis on strength and power work in a run training program seemed to many a misstep.

Often heralded as the inspiration for the 1970s running boom, Frank Shorter, the 1972 Olympic gold medalist in the marathon, was not just skinny—he was threadbare. The belief that running performance required carrying nothing but the absolute minimum in terms of muscle mass has been a constant theme in distance running.

Yet at a time when the American running boom was at full throttle and high-mileage, superskinny runners ruled the day, a study[4] was performed to determine the effects of weight training on the aerobic power development of distance runners. Would weight training add unnecessary weight and slow runners down? Would it waste energy that should be devoted exclusively to running?

In the 10-week study, not only did the strength work not diminish the runners' aerobic power, but VO_2max tests at the end of the 10 weeks showed a whopping 12 percent increase.

Still, criticism persists about runners using weights. Some coaches believe that it undercuts running economy, slows runners down, and injures them—or, at the very least, steals away time that would be better off spent running more miles.

Nevertheless, research has been supportive of runners incorporating strength work. As far as economy (how much running performance you exact from your intake of oxygen), a 1997 study split 12 runners into two groups, one adding full-body strength training to their program and the other sticking to just running.[5] The strength training group saw a 4 percent improvement in running economy over the purist group. A Finnish study recorded an 8 percent gain in running economy with runners using a 9-week explosive power program.[6]

To those who understand how the body adapts to different types of training stimulus, this is no surprise. Explosive movements engage the fast-twitch muscle fibers, which are responsible for generating quick speed, and also train the other muscle fibers to adopt some of the traits of the fast-twitch fibers. The result? Faster run times.

But what if you perform these weight training movements at high intensity, circuit training style? Won't you get hurt?

Quite the opposite, as it turns out. Coach Owen Anderson puts it bluntly: "An outstanding feature of circuit training is its relatively low injury rate, especially compared with running long distances."[7] In an indirect nod to CrossFit-style workouts, he adds, "Circuit-training sessions that incorporate a series of challenging exercises and drills carried out one after the other, without a significant break, can often push oxygen consumption rates up to 90 to 100 percent of VO_2max and heart rates above 90 percent of maximum" (see the "CrossFit Conditioning" sidebar, page 60).

This is especially important for older athletes. As we age, our bodies produce less testosterone and human growth hormone. The result is a gradual loss of muscle mass and speed. The aging process cannot be stopped, but it can be slowed down by engaging in various forms of strength training. That's one of the benefits of adopting the CFE method of training.

Another benefit derived from CFE training is improved balance and stability—not just in running but in all activities. That's because the complex movements used in CFE training establish neural connections between the brain and the skeletomuscular system that make complex movements more familiar and easier to handle. This opens the door not only to enjoying a greater range of sports and activities but also to maintaining an active, healthy lifestyle even into the senior years.

Finally, when considering the potential benefits of weight training and circuit training for runners, many people ask what the elite runners are doing. In fact, a growing number are using some form of ancillary strength training, but as stated at the beginning of this book, our intent is not to argue about the best path to becoming an elite runner. Rather, we hope to illuminate an alternative path that may be the right answer for those who have other goals, such as health and longevity in their running, and are looking for a way to get away from their injury patterns.

CROSSFIT CONDITIONING

I decided to put Owen Anderson's conclusions to the test, using my own body as the laboratory to determine how a high-intensitiy circuit training (HICT) workout or CrossFit workout can be used to train the energy systems in a way that boosts the anaerobic threshold and VO_2max.[11] In other words, in view of the evidence that a 7-minute HICT workout can stimulate similar adaptations to a low-intensity 90-minute run, I wanted to see the reflection of this intensity in my heart rate during a workout consisting of functional strength movements with no running.

Figure 3.1 shows the heart rate profile of a CrossFit "met-con" workout that I did on October 24, 2013. "Met-con" is short for "metabolic conditioning," a term indicating that stamina and endurance are pushed hard in the session. It was a high-repetition workout consisting of 4 sets of burpees and dumbbell snatches, in this repetition pattern: 24-12-6-24. There was no running involved.

I started off with 24 burpees, followed by 24 snatches, then immediately went to 12 burpees, 12 snatches, and so forth—with no significant break between sets. This yielded under 9 minutes of

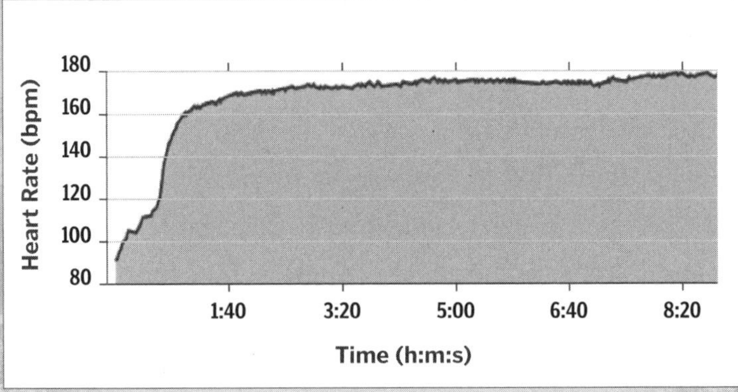

FIGURE 3.1: HEART RATE PROFILE FOR A METABOLIC CONDITIONING WORKOUT

functional fitness work, with a heavy draw on core muscles and various explosive power muscles.

As the figure indicates, my heart rate leaped to more than 160 beats per minute (bpm). For most of the workout, it was above 170 bpm and near 180 bpm. Within the context of the CFE model, I had relied on this workout to give me an effective endurance boost rather than relying on an easy LSD run.

A Close-up Look at Circuit Training

Although circuit training as a tool for distance runners has never been a mainstream concept, a study in the 1970s suggested its usefulness.[8] Twenty men and 20 women completed a circuit consisting of 10 exercises, including bench presses, back arches, leg presses, and back cable pull-downs.

Each exercise set was followed by a 15-second break, which kept the participants' heart rates at around 75 percent of their maximum. During the 10-week program, the participants did no running. Nevertheless, a follow-up test showed endurance improvements of 5 to 6 percent. More recent research has confirmed these results, showing that from a biochemical standpoint, an athlete can—with less than 10 minutes of high-intensity circuit work—achieve adaptations similar to if not better than those achieved through LSD workouts.

This conclusion was confirmed in a 2013 overview of the effect and value of circuit training workouts such as CrossFit by Chris Jordan, the director of exercise physiology at the Human Performance Institute in Orlando, Florida, who reviewed the research on high-intensity circuit training (HICT).[9] Jordan and his colleague Brett Klika examined studies suggesting that an HICT session can, within a matter of minutes, offer a training dose similar in effect to a long, low-intensity bout of traditional cardio exercise, such as riding a bike for 90 minutes.

Jordan and Klika wrote, "HICT is not a new concept, but it is growing in popularity because of its efficiency and practicality for a time-constrained society. The combination of aerobic and resistance training in a high-intensity, limited-rest design can deliver numerous health benefits in much less time than traditional programs."[10]

In an interview, Jordan told me of fitness gains similar to those MacKenzie experienced when he incorporated CrossFit workouts into his program: improvements in VO_2max, full-body strength gains, increased fat burning, decreased insulin resistance, and a powerful hormone response.

I asked Jordan what he thought of a distance runner replacing one or more of his or her weekly running workouts with an HICT workout. He believed this would be an excellent fit. "When we look at exercise, intensity and duration are the two important variables," Jordan says. "When intensity increases, duration can decrease. There's an opportunity to get the same benefits of a long workout in less time. There's research saying that we get even more results from the high-intensity/low-duration workout."

Getting Started

To follow the CFE training plans in this book, a runner can plug in visits to a CrossFit gym or perform CrossFit-style workouts at home. The best way to learn technique so that you can use the CFE training model is to join a CrossFit gym (or "box") and sign up for its beginner program, typically called an "on-ramp" program. These provide intensive instruction with low student-to-teacher ratios. Alternatively, Chapter 5 details two on-ramp programs that can be done at home.

In the mainstream media, CrossFit gyms have been depicted as modern-day torture chambers suitable only for crazed, obsessive athletes, but the reality is quite different. In the past four years, I've visited and trained in more than 30 different boxes across the country, and it's a rare class when I do not see a mix of ages and abilities, including middle-aged parents. (I, too, am a middle-aged parent.) As one CrossFit gym owner told me, safety and slow progression are everything to the successful CrossFit box. Boxes that develop reputations for pushing athletes too hard and too fast don't stay in business.

Do some investigative work to find a CrossFit gym that appeals to you, and sign up for the on-ramp program (see the "Choosing a Gym" sidebar, page 65). A coach will lead you toward developing a basic level of proficiency for the workouts.

How long will it take to learn the movements? Depending on age, athletic background, mobility issues, and injury history, among other factors, this may take just a month. Or it may take a number of months. The first time you try a thruster (a taxing combination of a front squat and overhead press into a single, explosive movement), an overhead squat, or a kipping pull-up (pull-ups with a gymnast's full-body kip move), you might think you're in over your head. That's what I thought, anyway. But if you remain humble, patient, and consistent, you will be surprised at how well your body responds.

As detailed in *Inside the Box*, I was in my late 40s and a limping wreck when I started CrossFit workouts, with such extreme restrictions in shoulder and hip mobility and such tight hamstrings that just about everything had to be scaled back so that I could participate. But that's what a good CrossFit gym and coach will do for you: help you scale things back so you can get started, get some traction, and make the strength and mobility improvements that will enable you to do higher-level workouts.

My advice to runners like me? Join a CrossFit gym at least for the first two months. Even the movements that appear to be simple—such as an air squat—in reality are difficult to learn on your own. A good coach will watch you carefully and cue you away from mistakes and bad movement patterns.

For those wishing to do the workouts at home, the following guide will help you get started.

Going It Alone

The training plans included in this book are set up so that a newcomer to CFE can get started with some basic body-weight movements and introductory CrossFit-style workouts.

Learning the fundamental movements on your own can be tricky, especially if you are new to strength training. You may have an iPad or a book propped up in front of you as you try to replicate an air squat, but errors are easy to make: The knees cave in, the depth of the squat is insufficient, the lower lumbar curve is lost. Without a coach giving you educated feedback and assistance, it's challenging to correctly learn and execute even the most basic of CrossFit movements.

One excellent option for performing the CrossFit workouts at home is to find a committed training partner who can be your eyes while you are trying to fulfill the requirements of good form. If you have to go "lone wolf" on this, shooting video of yourself as you try out the movements is helpful. The key thing to remember is that you can't trust your mind's eye—it may feel like you're doing it right, but you need to get confirmation and feedback.

CHOOSING A GYM

So how does one take up CrossFit Endurance, anyway? A conventional running plan is simple to read and follow. It's usually just running. But CFE involves strength and conditioning movements plucked from the worlds of gymnastics, Olympic lifting, and strength training, with many of the exercises requiring proper form for both safety and efficacy.

Can you do CFE alone? Yes, and along with the training schedules presented in this book, we give you a list of the more accessible movements and workouts that can be fit into the program with a minimum of equipment.

That said, we highly recommend joining a CrossFit gym and having a coach usher you through at least the first 2 months of your exposure to functional strength workouts. Some CrossFit gyms even have specially trained CFE coaches and groups with which you can train. You can work with a group performing the CrossFit workouts in the gym and also train with one another on the road or at the track.

If you can't find a CrossFit gym with a CFE-specific program and you still want guidance through the strength workouts, the training plans included in this book are designed so that you can carry out the running workouts on your own and drop into a CrossFit box for those workouts.

The most valuable thing you can do to ensure success if you join a CrossFit affiliate is to be extremely picky about the gym you choose. Do your homework, visit as many gyms as you can, and try to interview the coaches.

The CrossFit affiliate system is not like a Starbucks franchise system, where everything looks, feels, and works the same way. Each box has a different personality, and there can be bias in the programming.

CONTINUED

CONTINUED

I asked Dr. Leon Chang, an MD and co-owner of CrossFit Elysium in San Diego, what advice he could offer on choosing a box. He gave the following recommendations.

FIND THE LICENSED CROSSFIT BOXES IN YOUR AREA. Chang warns people to keep clear of the various rip-offs of the CrossFit model. CrossFit.com provides a list of nearly 10,000 certified affiliates worldwide.

NARROW THE LIST. "Inevitably, there will be some great affiliates and coaches out there, and some not-so-great ones," Chang says. "Be your own best advocate in selecting the best gym for you. Talk to the coaches and get a feel for what they stand for." Do they seem to generally care about your health and you as a person? Or do you simply represent another monthly check?

CHECK OUT THE PROGRAMMING. When interviewing the coaches at a box, ask them how they plan the workouts. "The coaches should be able to tell you why each workout is programmed and what the overall training effect—both short-term and long-term—is intended to be," Chang says. "If they can't do that, they probably don't know what they're doing."

Another variable to help you narrow this list is to ask about how a runner might fit into the box's programming. For a list of boxes that offer CFE programs, go to CrossFitEndurance.com.

TRY OUT A CLASS. Many CrossFit affiliates offer an introductory workout at no cost or a community workout where you can get a feel for the training and for the culture. Chang recommends these as good opportunities to see how committed the coaches are to the needs and skills of their membership. What you're looking for are coaches who are absolutely obsessed with quality execution of the exercises.

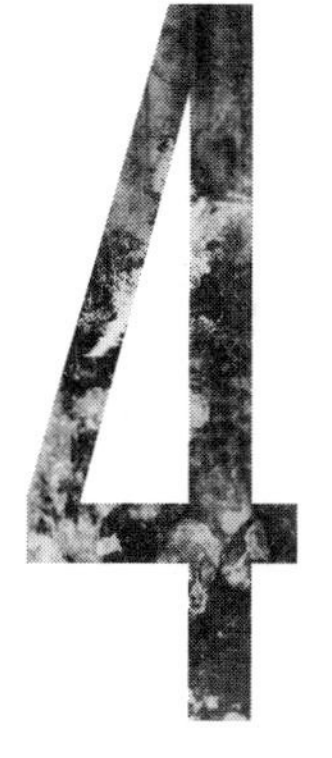

NUTRITION THE CROSSFIT ENDURANCE WAY

More important than what you eat in a competition is refining how you eat day to day, something that becomes easier the more we make good choices in eating.

—MARK ALLEN, SIX-TIME HAWAII IRONMAN CHAMPION

In the CrossFit Endurance world, the conceit that runners can eat whatever they want—because they just burn it off—does not exist. Rather, good nutrition is a high priority and is considered essential to health, longevity, performance, tissue repair, and hormonal balance.

For decades, runners have striven to keep their glycogen stores filled to the brim. Nutritionists, coaches, books, and magazines have egged them on in this pursuit. At a road race, runners wash down bagels with a high-carb sports drink before a race and suck on 100-calorie gel packets during the race. You'll even see runners using gels in short races, such as 5K road races, although such events are not nearly long enough for a runner to burn through the body's glycogen reserves.

Runners were encouraged to choose a high-carbohydrate, low-fat, low-protein diet such as the Pritikin Diet, which was the buzz diet of the 1980s.

Recommendations of a high-carbohydrate diet weren't restricted to fad diets, however. Until recently, the USDA Food Pyramid (see Figure 4.1) encouraged all Americans to treat the "bread, cereal, rice and pasta" group as the foundation of their eating. A diet high in processed carbohydrates was implied to be a healthy diet. (The new "Choose My Plate" diagram, Figure 4.2, adopted by the USDA in 2011, divides the plate into vegetables, fruits, protein, and grains—pretty much in quarters—with dairy off to the side in a small bowl.)

For the distance runner burning 500-plus calories per run and more than 2,500 calories in a marathon, the implication was clear: more pasta, more bread, and more calories from carbohydrate. This

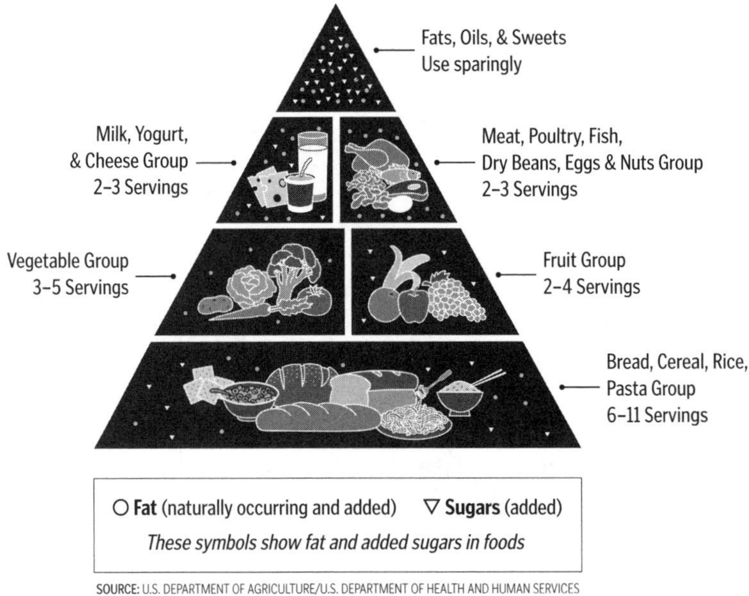

FIGURE 4.1: USDA FOOD GUIDE PYRAMID

obsession with carbohydrate replenishment and loading in the running world is epitomized by the traditional pre-race pasta dinner held by many road races across the country, as well as the tables loaded with carbohydrates lined up for runners after a race, which typically include items such as bananas, cookies, sports drinks, and sports bars.

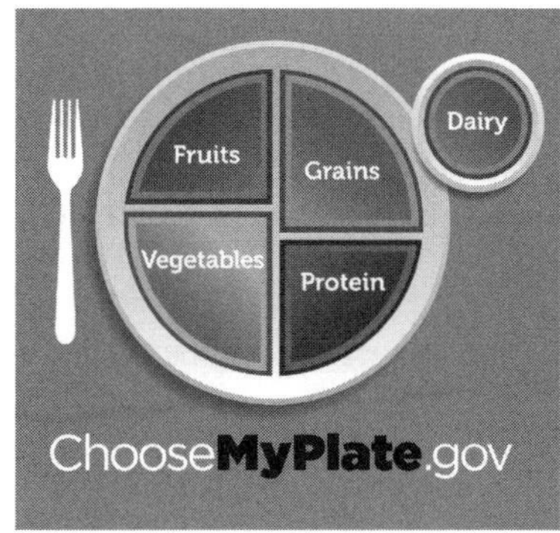

FIGURE 4.2: USDA "CHOOSE MY PLATE" DIAGRAM

The rationale behind these carb-fests went like this: You're a runner burning fuel. Fuel is carbohydrate, and your body stores carbs in the form of glycogen. Your body can store about 2,000 calories' worth of glycogen in the muscles and liver, so a runner should keep pumping in more carbs as energy for the muscles, either directly into the bloodstream or by refilling glycogen where it is stored, in the liver.

The runner failing to attend to this suggested pattern of fueling and refueling was warned that he or she might "hit the wall," or "bonk"—or, worse, fail to recover adequately from training and racing and expose him- or herself to the risk of overtraining or getting injured. Within this fueling strategy, the belief that your body could rely primarily on fat burning was cast to the margins.

With all these recommendations coming from the USDA and the running establishment during the 1980s through the 1990s and beyond, it's easy to understand why that traditional pre-race pasta party appealed to the average runner. But things have changed since the turn of the century, especially regarding our understanding of the consequences of a high-carb diet. The discussion—often emotionally heated, as discussions of diet seem to be—has brought to light a new question: What is the hormonal impact of the meal you just ate? Specifically, what is the insulin response?

The problem with a diet that gets most of its calories from high-carb, processed foods is that it often relies on high-fructose corn syrup (aka refined sugar) for taste and is high on the glycemic index, which measures the rate at which foods are processed by the body and converted into glycogen, or blood sugar.

The consequence of this kind of diet is that when we continually dump loads of sugar into the bloodstream, our bodies struggle to process and store this bonanza. To accomplish this, the body releases more and more insulin, which is a hormone that transports sugar to the liver and throughout the body. Over time, this system becomes overloaded, and we become insulin-resistant. If a fasting blood test reveals that you have a high amount of glucose in the blood, it's a sign that you've developed insulin resistance.

Achieving your athletic potential requires scrutiny of exactly how you are fueling your body.

This is where the discussion can get swamped with arcane terminology. Terms like "hyperglycemia," "metabolic syndrome," and "cellular inflammation" get thrown around, but they all point to one result: a growing insulin resistance is a step toward the early stages of type 2 diabetes, which can lead to kidney failure and heart disease.

With this in mind, in February 2009, the American Heart Association—in consultation with Dr. Robert Lustig, a specialist in hormone disorders and a leading academic voice against the evils of processed sugar—released dietary guidelines that advocated cutting down on sugar consumption. However, many runners have held on to the belief that as long as you're putting in your weekly mileage, you can eat pretty much whatever you want without consequence.

I've been guilty of this assumption myself. Once a year my friends and I used to engage in a flagrant demonstration of the concept with what we called "the Donut Run," in which we would crisscross San Francisco, from Happy Donuts to All-Star Donuts and more—eating a donut at each stop.

But research has shown that runners are not immune to the effects of sugar dumping. A March 2014 article in the *Wall Street Journal* titled "Why Runners Can't Eat Whatever They Want" described research studies that have shown lifelong runners developing coronary plaque.[1] The article was triggered by the plight of prominent runner and Boston Marathon race director Dave McGillivray, who had recently been diagnosed with heart disease. The most recent study cited in the article revealed that runners who had run at least one marathon a year for 25 years had, on average, more coronary plaque buildup in their arterial walls than a group of sedentary men.[2]

As Paul Thompson, a marathoner and the chief of cardiology at Hartford Hospital, told the *Wall Street Journal*, the cavalier attitude of "I will run it off" is common among marathoners, "almost sometimes to an arrogance."

Although the research mentioned in the article hasn't yet identified the actual culprit—diet? too much running?—it stands to reason that until conclusive data are collected to establish the cause for the coronary plaque, making a high-quality diet a higher priority in a runner's life seems prudent.

One internationally recognized endurance nutrition expert, Dr. John Ivy at the University of Texas, told me in an interview that his research indicates that although a runner's exercise activity may cloak the negative effects of a bad diet, that doesn't mean there is no harm occurring on a metabolic level. When runners are forced to stop running, Ivy said, they can start showing signs of being prediabetic within a matter of days.

In other words, if runners think they can get away with a junk diet because they will just burn anything and everything by running a lot, they need to think again; there may be consequences brewing below the surface.

Diet and Nutrition: Critical to High Performance?

Brian MacKenzie long ago shed the stereotypical runner's view of food. For an early interview with him, we met at his house in Costa Mesa, California. The kitchen had a laboratory vibe to it. He had a freezer stocked with grass-fed beef and metallic bottles of fish oil. For lunch, he sautéed several cups of locally grown produce and added some organic free-range chicken. He drank fizzy water, and after a workout in his garage gym, he offered me a bottle of coconut water with grass-fed whey protein mixed in.

I found it impossible not to ask him why he was doing all this. Why all the fuss with diet?

In the CrossFit Endurance model, nutrition is the foundation to health; it is critical to supporting all of the bodily functions. If your nutrition is not right, you may progress as an athlete, but not as far as you can if your diet is a front-burner priority.

An example supporting MacKenzie's point comes from the story of American runner Anthony Famiglietti. Despite growing up on a diet that a nutritionist would consider junk-food malnourishment—the closest thing to a vegetable that he consumed was reportedly pizza sauce—Famiglietti was a three-time national champion in the 3000-meter steeplechase and won gold in the World University Games in 2001.

In 2007, Famiglietti was 26 years old and still an ardent patron of the fast-food industry when he won the USA 5K road race title along with collecting personal records across a range of distances. However, things fell to pieces for Famiglietti in 2008. After a disappointing steeplechase finish at the USA nationals, his body revolted. According to Matt Fitzgerald, who wrote an article on Famiglietti for Competitor.com, "For the next two weeks he could not even run a full mile without a walking break. It was then that he decided to finally find out what broccoli tastes like."[3]

According to Fitzgerald, Famiglietti gave up what had been his staples well into adulthood (fast-food burgers, frozen pizza, and candy) and made unprocessed foods such as fruits, vegetables, and fish his main source of fuel. In 2008, he won the steeplechase at the USA Olympic trials and recorded his personal best at the Beijing Games.

It is hard to say definitively why Famiglietti experienced his breakdown and later success. Was it his dietary shift? Given how poor his diet was to begin with and the changes he adopted to correct for it, it is highly probable that nutrition played a major role. The adage "quality in, quality out" seems to apply. The widespread view that all calories are the same, and that as long as you're getting the right amount of calories you're good to go, is rejected by the CFE model.

Let's return to the stored-fuel situation a runner faces. A runner can store 400 to 500 grams of carbs in his or her muscles and liver, or approximately 2,000 calories' worth of energy.

The carb-fueled runner model hinges on the idea that stored body fat is a relatively inefficient source to process, despite the enormous reserves: Approximately 40,000 calories of energy are stored in the body fat of even the fittest of athletes. Runners and running coaches have operated under the principle that one adaptation that occurs through training is that our bodies learn to burn fat more efficiently, but there are limits. By all means, rev up your fat-burning efficiency as much as you can with training, but carbohydrates are easier to burn, and therefore they are often considered the superior energy source.

Here's how it works: While a gram of carbohydrate can be directly converted into 4 calories of the primary currency of energy—adenosine triphosphate (ATP)—through a process called glycogenolysis, burning fat is more complicated. A gram of fat offers up 9 calories of energy when converted to ATP through lipolysis, but because of fat's steeper carbon-to-oxygen ratio, the body's oxygen use goes up.

Consequently, fat is generally considered the more cumbersome of energy sources. Imagine that you were stranded in the Arctic and had a woodpile, on the one hand, and a drum of uranium, on the other. The woodpile (which represents carbs in this example) is an easy-to-use source of fuel that could keep you warm for a couple of hours. To use the uranium (which represents fat), you would have to purify it and do all sorts of things to turn it into a useful form of heat, but it would supply you with enough heat to stay warm for a much longer time.

As Brian MacKenzie realized years ago, a glaring worry for carb-obsessed runners, particularly those specializing in the marathon distance and beyond, is that the reliance on carbs during a race can require a constant stream of simple sugars, bringing with it wild spikes and drops in blood sugar levels. With a tank capacity of 2,000 calories and suboptimal capacity to burn fat, the carb-dependent distance runner, both in long training runs and in races, is going to wreak a lot of insulin havoc on his or her body.

For long-term good health and performance, for runners and non-runners alike, the consequences of a high-carb diet simply must be taken into account.

Moving Toward a New Model of Nutrition

In recent years, scientists, coaches, and runners have been looking into more direct approaches toward improving the fat-burning efficiency of the human body during exercise. A 2011 study compared two groups of cyclists who were training for a 1-hour time trial.[4] One group ate a high-carb breakfast before training, and the other group did the same workout but prior to eating breakfast, while in a fasting state.

Although both groups showed equal improvement in the time trial, the group that fasted before workouts demonstrated increased fat-burning efficiency across a range of paces that their counterparts did not achieve. The implication? The fat-burner cyclists would be less likely to hit the wall in long workouts or races.

Jeff Volek and Stephen Phinney are scientists and authors interested in the possibilities of training the body to become more adept at burning fat. In their book *The Art and Science of Low Carbohydrate Performance*,[5] they argue that by following an aggressive low-carb diet over the course of several weeks, an endurance athlete lowers inflammation levels across the board and achieves accelerated fat-burning capacity.

These two reasons—better health prospects through a low-inflammation diet and being able to access greater stores of energy—prompted MacKenzie to be an early adopter of a low-carb, low-inflammation diet.

Much of what MacKenzie advocates is in sync with the "Paleo diet"—a mode of eating that is based on the idea that the digestive machinery of the human species as it has currently evolved isn't really that different than that of our cavemen ancestors, and thus we should eat accordingly. But MacKenzie's system is not as simple as that. He stresses that there is a lot of individual variation in nutrition and that what might be suitable for one runner might not work for another runner.

Still, there are at least two things that all runners should agree on, according to MacKenzie: avoiding foods that cause inflammation and choosing foods that are anti-inflammatory. To achieve these ends, the basic dietary prescription for a CFE athlete can be summed up in two simple and related ideas:

- *Shop the perimeter of the grocery store:* The interior shelves of most supermarkets hold countless boxes and cans of processed foods, many of which contain high-fructose corn syrup and vegetable oil. These ingredients not only are cheap but also allow these packages to sit on the shelves for long periods of time, which compromises the foods' nutritional value. Hence, MacKenzie advises runners to stick to the produce section and the meat, fish, and poultry sections of the store, which are typically located around the perimeter.

- *Eat real food:* Avoid processed food, and choose an organic variety whenever possible. Distance yourself from anything that originates from a factory farm.

For more detailed suggestions, MacKenzie offers this list of guidelines:

- *Meat*: Eat grass-fed beef and avoid grain-fed beef. (Grass-fed beef has more healthy fats—omega-3s—and fewer unhealthy fats than grain-fed beef.)[6]
- *Fish*: Choose wild-caught fish, and avoid factory farm fish. (Farmed salmon, for example, have fewer omega-3 fatty acids than wild-caught salmon).[7]
- *Vegetables and fruits:* Eat a lot of vegetables and some fruits, choosing seasonal and organic varieties when possible.
- *Dairy, legumes, grains, sugars, and sugar substitutes*: Avoid them. MacKenzie isn't a hard-liner on these; rather, his advice is that if you want optimal health and performance, try living without these foods for a while, allowing your body to reset itself, and see how you feel and perform. In one way or another, in the CFE view, all of these foods cause some distress to the body, whether it is through elevated inflammation, gastric distress, or insulin spikes. For objective information, get blood panels—particularly markers for cellular inflammation, such as C-reactive protein—done and have them rechecked after 6 weeks or so. If these dietary changes are making a difference, you might be compelled to stick with them.
- *Water*: Drink a lot of it, the equivalent of at least half your body weight in ounces every day.

The primary message MacKenzie has for runners is that achieving your athletic potential requires scrutiny of exactly how you are fueling your body. After all, would you want to pour moonshine into a Formula 1 race car? To the human engine and all the intricate systems that support it, a calorie is not just a calorie; the foods you choose can greatly impact your health and performance. If that race goal you've set for yourself really matters, it's time to consider every meal a factor in your success.

Mackenzie's Take on Nutrition: Be Your Own Lab Rat

"We always want to address nutrition in our athletes," Brian MacKenzie says, speaking about how he believes nutrition should be one of the highest priorities for a runner.

He is not a zealot for a particular diet, however, be it the Paleo diet or the high-fat/super-low-carb ketogenic diet. Instead, he advocates a general approach rather than one specific plan. As he explains, "Runners committed to achieving higher athletic performance with diet should be conducting an ongoing experiment to see what foods and meals work best for them on an individual basis."

For example, the genetics of a certain athlete may be such that a strict Paleo diet—which doesn't allow consumption of grains, legumes, or dairy—isn't necessary. If you have no problem digesting milk and don't notice any negative effects on your health or performance, MacKenzie sees no reason why you shouldn't drink milk. You will not know this, however, unless you are willing to get blood work done, remove milk from your diet for a period, and then have blood work redone. Then, if you believe the milk had no ill effect, slowly adding it back in is the only way you will know how your body handles it.

Implicit in this experimentation, however, is that you initially need to reset your body by following an extremely clean diet free of processed foods—a strict Paleo diet. After a period of adaptation, you can reintroduce a food such as milk or black beans and then pay attention to how your body reacts, monitoring energy levels, stomach comfort, performance in workouts, sleep quality, and the like. If there's no detrimental reaction, then the food gets a pass. The same sort of testing process would be employed to determine ideal quantities of the food, proportions of macronutrients in a meal, meal timing, and more. Some individuals may even thrive on a vegetarian diet, but they have to be willing to experiment to determine how such a diet affects their performance.

According to MacKenzie, "Runners committed to achieving higher athletic performance with diet should be conducting an ongoing experiment to see what foods and meals work best for them on an individual basis." This is where he sees a lot of people go wrong. "There is a serious lack of willingness to experiment in the world of nutrition, and I have been there too. When we play around with one way of eating and get some results with this new method, we fall too easily into the assumption this is the only way to eat." We become less willing to experiment, thereby missing the chance to find out if something else could work even better.

This, in short, is how MacKenzie coaches an athlete in regard to nutrition. It starts with the athlete keeping a food log for three days.

"The log gives us a good snapshot," MacKenzie says. "But from there, you have to be willing to play with the prescription to see what works best. The allegiance is not to a specific diet but to health and performance."

Following this phase, experimentation with different dietary prescriptions commences. Any mysteries that need solving are often attacked with the aid of blood testing, saliva tests, and urine tests. Digestion problems can also be sorted out with medical tests conducted on stool. Based on the collected data, the diet is tweaked, and eventually the athlete is retested.

MacKenzie's longest-running dietary lab rat is himself. A decade ago, his own diet was not unlike the standard high-carbohydrate diet that is often recommended for endurance athletes. But when he wanted to address problems with overly long recovery times and feeling generally cruddy, he started experimenting with lowering his carbohydrate intake.

What is the point of lower carbohydrate intake? The thesis that too much dietary carbohydrate leads to elevated blood sugar levels as it is digested, which is bad for health and athletic performance, was explored by Dr. Barry Sears in his Zone Diet books in the 1990s. The response from the mainstream nutrition world was mixed. But in the past 10 years, advocates for lowering sugar consumption have emerged. Dr. Robert Lustig, an endocrinologist at the University of California, and nutrition author Gary Taubes have been leading advocates for the notion that high sugar consumption overstimulates the body's insulin response, leading to obesity, diabetes, and other diseases.

MacKenzie's obsession is not only with health but also with athletic performance, and his personal dietary experiments continue to this day. A snapshot of MacKenzie's working diet looks something like this. Broadly, he follows the Paleo diet in terms of food choices: primarily grass-fed beef and an array of other organic meats, vegetables, some fruit, and monounsaturated fats from foods such as avocados and olive oil.

Recently, MacKenzie has been playing with different macronutrient ratios at different times of the day, with one of his key goals being to activate a reliance on burning stored body fat as opposed to stored carbohydrate. For breakfast, MacKenzie likes a high-protein/high-fat/low-carb mix: three eggs mixed with a large serving of arugula, avocado, and olive oil, with several slices of prosciutto.

Lunch is another low-carb meal, consisting of a salad along with some type of animal protein and more monounsaturated fats.

At dinner, MacKenzie increases his carb intake with sweet potato or squash in tandem with more animal protein. If he has a longer run or bike ride planned for the following day, the amount of carbs will be higher. Following a high-intensity/moderate-duration stamina workout—called a "met-con" in the CrossFit world, short for "metabolic conditioning"—or run session, he makes sure to consume carbohydrate to enhance recovery. This has all been learned through an ordeal of trial and much error. Quite a few high-intensity, moderate-duration sessions were followed by inadequate carbohydrate intake, and MacKenzie realized that recovery was insufficient under those conditions.

Variety is central to the "animal protein" component of MacKenzie's diet. Some of his more exotic selections include elk, buffalo, wild boar, ostrich, and kangaroo meat. He's also slowly adding organ meats—which he says are unpopular in the United States but not uncommon within European gastronomy. "If you're going to eat Paleo," he asserts, "then eating organ meats is in line with how our ancestors ate." The point being, when cavemen managed to kill a beast for dinner, they ate everything that was potentially edible. But MacKenzie says that his own reason for choosing organ meats is their high nutrient density.

MacKenzie's diet includes a sports drink of his own creation that includes a long-chain starch shown to boost fat utilization.[8] He also takes fish oil on a regular basis, although he has begun to "cycle" it rather than take it every day. MacKenzie has noticed that the jolt of accelerated recovery provided by omega-3 fatty acids (which are contained in fish oil) drops off if he takes the oil on a daily basis. His observation is that the body adapts to it. "Two days on, one day off seems to be a good cycle," he says.

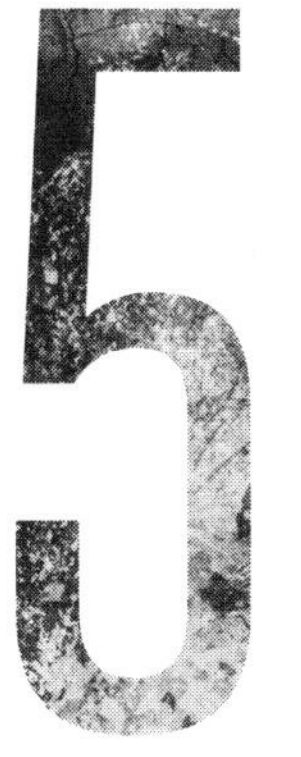

CROSSFIT ENDURANCE: INTRODUCING YOUR WORKOUT BUILDING BLOCKS

One thing we've consistently seen with those moving from traditional programs into CFE is that their pain tolerance goes through the roof.

—BRIAN MACKENZIE

The CrossFit Endurance running method organizes your training such that, once you understand it, you are the creator and master of your race preparation plan.

In this chapter, we present a transition plan for the traditional runner to get you up to speed and comfortable with the CrossFit piece of the training equation. Later in the chapter, we provide a list of slightly more advanced CrossFit workouts that you can plug into your race-specific training plans when a CrossFit workout is called for.

CrossFit as a Diagnostic Tool

Are CrossFit workouts valuable for runners because they improve strength, power, and conditioning? Absolutely. A less obvious but no less important value of CrossFit workouts for runners is the way in which they function as a diagnostic tool.

One of the great values in performing the exercises and workouts in CrossFit is that they will cast a spotlight on problems long before any show up as overuse injuries. Weaknesses, imbalances, and range-of-motion issues that might not be apparent to a coach during a running workout can become visible when you perform squats with a loaded barbell or attempt to do handstand push-ups. Better to catch these deficiencies sooner than later, before they work their way to the surface.

Whether you are a beginning runner or a star athlete, CrossFit workouts can reveal athletic shortcomings. Lateral wobbles show that your hip stabilizers aren't doing their job, and wobbly knees reveal quads that aren't performing to their potential. Lapses in form, or failure to successfully complete the assigned workout, will indicate a problem that CFE can then help you address and correct.

Indeed, CrossFit is, by definition, a general strength and conditioning program, designed to expose an athlete to a spectrum of athletic training challenges, including speed, power, coordination, flexibility, balance, agility, strength, accuracy, stamina, and cardiovascular endurance. A series of CrossFit workouts, using everything from gymnastics movements to Olympic lifts, is designed to tax an athlete in each of these categories.

While a classically trained distance runner will excel in the cardiovascular aspect of a CFE workout, he or she will likely have trouble with the CFE workouts that emphasize power, agility, or flexibility. However, as MacKenzie advises runners, don't get frustrated if you discover that you have some holes in your fitness.

At first, you may experience difficulty, for example, jumping up onto a 24-inch plyometric box. But don't look on that difficulty as a failure. Rather, because your goal is to build your capacity to jump—which requires a combination of power, flexibility, balance, coordination, and stamina—this discovery provides vital opportunities for you to harvest additional running performance.

In order to scale back the exercise, you may have to start with a 12-inch box, which looks ridiculously low compared with what others in a CrossFit workout might be using. Be prepared to check your ego at the door and accept—and even enjoy—being a beginner. Be assured that results come quickly as long as you attack your weaknesses with consistent work and dedication. The fruits of your labor will follow: more speed, more endurance, and a lowered risk of injury.

As you integrate CrossFit exercises and workouts into your program, along with the recommended skill and drill work, think of yourself as the head engineer of a power plant. Your job is to constantly scan the plant for any weaknesses in the flow of power or any instability in the systems.

One of the great values in performing the exercises and workouts in CrossFit is that they will cast a spotlight on problems long before any show up as overuse injuries.

This isn't an overnight process. But over the course of months, you'll reap the benefits as you begin to burn calories as efficiently as possible while you fly down the road.

One of the critical principles at the core of CrossFit is variety. To stimulate the most benefit, the athlete should avoid routine workout patterns that lull the body into staleness. Fortunately, there's no limit to the possible combinations of movements that constitute a good CrossFit workout.

However, one limiting factor for the beginner—especially a long-time runner who has not performed much in the way of strength, conditioning, and range-of-motion work—is an inadequate amount of mobility, coordination, and experience to perform the more advanced exercises in a CrossFit program. Ask any experienced CrossFit coach about the initial weeks of working with a runner. Runners tend to bring tremendous drive and mental toughness, but when it comes to basic movements, they are hampered by poor range of motion in their hips, ankles, and shoulders. That is because of the short and choppy nature of the running motion, which is repeated thousands of times in each running workout.

> Over the course of months, you'll reap the benefits as you begin to burn calories as efficiently as possible while you fly down the road.

CrossFit is the antidote to these problems. A beginner can achieve tremendous gains in strength, power, and mobility using even the most basic movements. Even if the beginner limits his or her CrossFit workouts to movements using push-ups, burpees, air squats, and pull-ups—with the emphasis on performing the workouts correctly rather than quickly—training benefits will come fast and furious.

The best path for a runner unfamiliar with this brand of training is working with a knowledgeable coach at a good CrossFit facility. But, as we'll discuss, this program is also designed for those without access to such facilities and coaches. Ask a U.S. marine with a CrossFit background about doing CrossFit in a remote location in Afghanistan, and he or she will likely describe how fit it is possible to get using a sandbag and a jump rope.

For the traditional runner who has had minimal exposure to strength and conditioning work, it may be hard to imagine adding exercises such as overhead squats, box jumps, and clean and jerks to your workout regimen. Maybe the equipment or logistics seems overwhelming.

Not the case. Adding CrossFit workouts to your program—whether in a CrossFit gym or in your own home—is easier than you think. In this chapter, we'll begin by presenting a 6-week program to simply introduce CrossFit into your routine. Next we'll review the drills and exercises you will use within this transition program (as well as in the race-training programs in Chapter 6). Then we will list CFE exercises that can be plugged into the race-specific CrossFit Endurance programs that are provided in Chapter 6. Finally, we will look at the importance of recovery.

Before we get started, let's review the key terms and abbreviations that you'll see in the CFE programs.

- *AMRAP: as many rounds as possible.* The aim is to perform as many rounds and as many reps as possible—with good form—within the given time. Record your number of rounds and extra reps in your log to keep track of your progress.

- *Cadence training.* "Cadence" refers to stride rate. The ideal cadence is 180 steps per minute (meaning that each foot touches the ground 90 times per minute). To track your cadence, set a small electronic metronome at 180 and match the beat. When you start working on cadence, it can seem hard to sustain, but after you've exposed your nervous system and muscles to the faster pattern for a while, the new faster stride rate will come to feel natural.

- *NFT: not for time.* Complete the workout at your own pace, emphasizing good form.
- *FT: for time.* Record the time it takes you to perform the workout, and record it in your log to track your progress.
- *WR: walk recovery.*
- *Tabata sprints:* The Tabata protocol consists of 20 seconds of hard training followed by 10 seconds of rest, for a total of 8 rounds. It has been shown to produce substantial VO_2max (that is, oxygen uptake) increases with just a 4-minute workout. It can be performed on a track or a straight stretch of road, or on a treadmill, using an elevated grade to increase the workload. MacKenzie's athletes use a treadmill to work up to a 12 percent grade and run at 5K race pace.
- *Time trial (TT):* a measurement of maximum work capacity/power output over a set amount of time or distance. TTs give information on your current running fitness and allow you to better dial in the best paces for your interval and tempo workouts. A TT is also effective training on its own. Treat one as you would a race—take time to warm up, starting with drills and working your way up to striders and sprints to ensure that your engine is hot. Cool down with the same level of focus, giving attention to slow running and stretching. This helps prevent injury and gives your circulatory and lymphatic systems time to clear out waste products.

To watch videos of each of the drills and exercises presented in this book, go to the web site unbreakablerunner.com.

Drills

The training plans call for drills along with each workout. They are designed to help you work on skill and stability. Developing running skill and midline stability is central to the CFE philosophy, so make sure that you don't skip any of these drills.

On training days when your program calls for you to perform drills, follow this checklist:

- ☐ *Hollow rock:* 3 × 10 or 1- to 2-minute hold in correct hollow position.
- ☐ *Hop with forward lean:* 3 × 3 to 5.
- ☐ *Pulling wall:* 3 × 20 with each foot.
- ☐ *Alternating foot pull:* 3 × 5 to 10 on the right, then 5 to 10 on the left.
- ☐ *Fast runs:* The length depends on the work set. If the work set is 200s, start with 2 × 100 meters at 80 to 90 percent effort, follow that with 2 × 200 meters at greater than 90 percent effort, then start the work set. Rest as needed between sets.

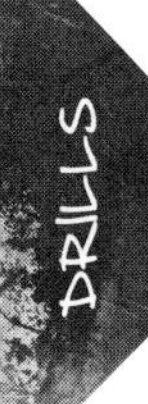

Hollow Rock

Hollow rock develops trunk strength and midline stabilization, which allows runners to hold good form even when they are fatigued at the end of a long race.

Lie faceup on the ground with arms reaching overhead. Tighten up your muscles—including abs and glutes—and imagine that you're trying to pin your belly button to your spine. You should be aiming to achieve a shape like a crescent moon, with your lower back flat on the ground and your arms and legs elevated about a foot off the ground. Now use your legs to kick and power a rocking-chair motion.

SCALE: If you have a weak core, this exercise is tough to do properly at first. Build up strength by first spending time holding planks and using other traditional trunk strength exercises. You can also scale hollow rock by holding the engaged position without progressing into the rocking motion.

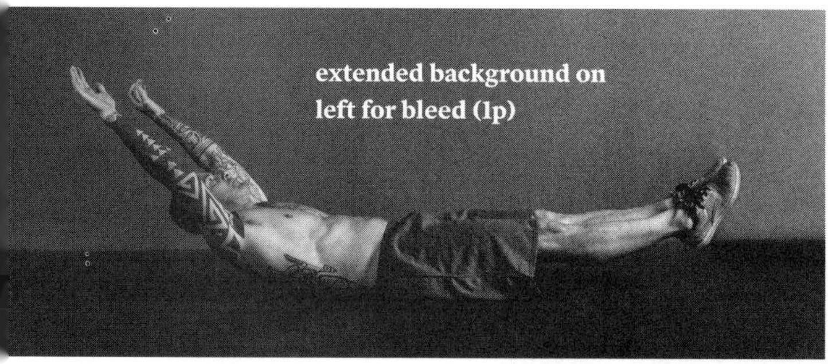

extended background on left for bleed (1p)

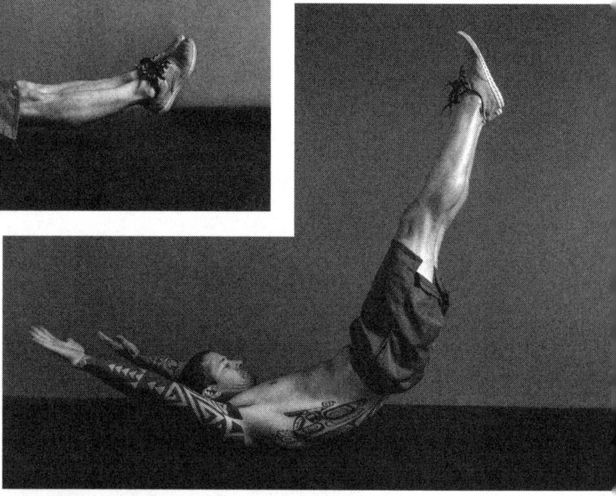

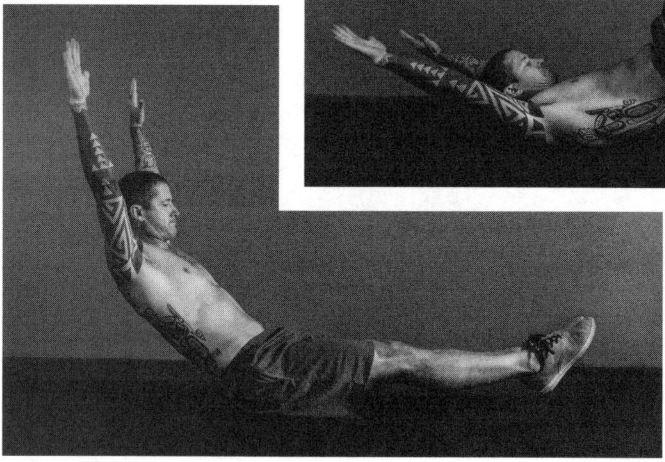

Hop with Forward Lean

This drill will help teach you how to properly use gravity with a falling forward lean. It transitions runners to a more compact stride; instead of reaching out with the leg and landing on the heel, midline stability is maintained and the hips become more central to the flow of power.

Begin with small vertical hops, as if jumping rope, engaging the core. Once you are hopping, allow your body to fall forward, hinging from the ankles instead of the waist. Continue to hop as you allow gravity to move you forward. Imagine that you are a pogo stick; focus on the elasticity in your feet and ankles to propel you. Lean for 3 to 5 hops without scuffing the feet, and then level out for 3 more hops.

SCALE: Practice leaning and squatting without actually hopping, which will accustom you to the movement and build strength in your hips and quads.

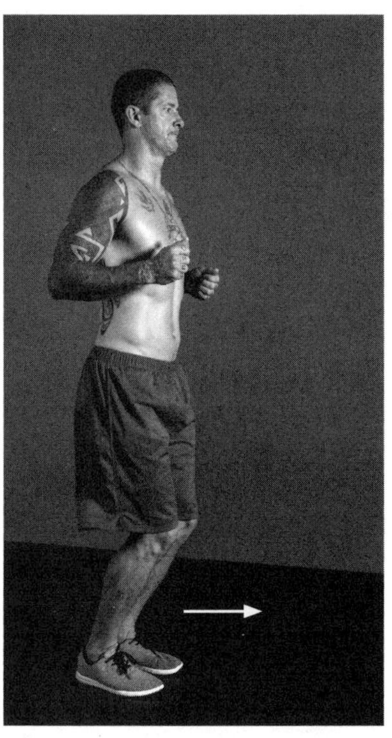

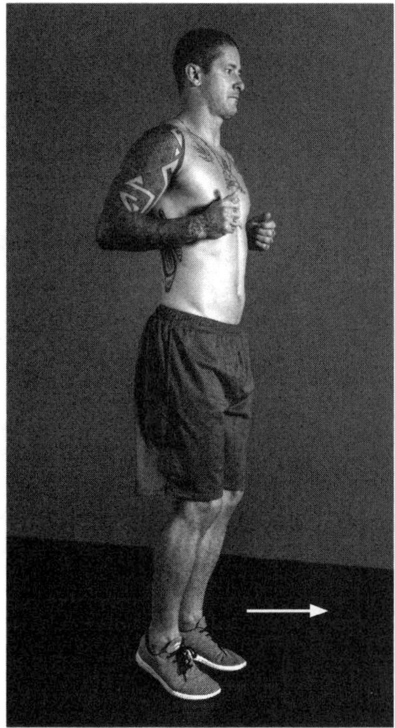

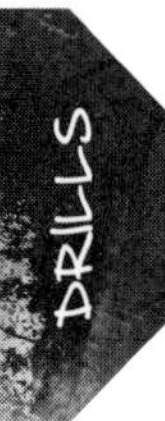

Pulling Wall

The primary goal of this drill is to learn how to activate your hamstrings and glutes when pulling the foot up from the ground after landing.

Stand 6 inches away from a wall and engage your core. Now practice pulling your foot up from the ground directly beneath your hip, using a light but quick snapping motion initiated by the hamstring. Use the wall to keep your foot from extending too far behind you.

Do 20 reps with each leg while focusing on using your hamstring and glutes to do the work. For runners who have relied more on their hip flexors than their hamstrings to run, this exercise will wake up some dormant tissue—you may even cramp up a bit. You'll want the hamstring activation to translate into your running, with a quick popping off the ground with each foot pull.

SCALE: Start with 5 pulls on each leg, and slowly add repetitions with each workout until you can do 20.

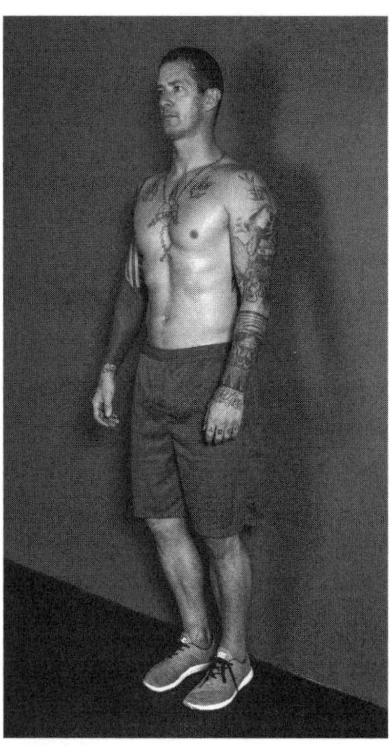

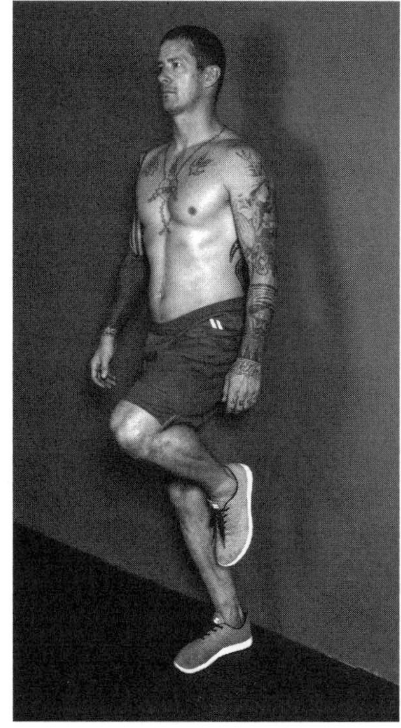

Alternating Foot Pull

This drill follows mastery of the pulling wall drill. Rather than jackhammering away with one foot, alternate each foot as you do when you're running. Take this movement into your striders and other warm-up running drills.

SCALE: Instead of alternating with each step, alternate every 5 steps.

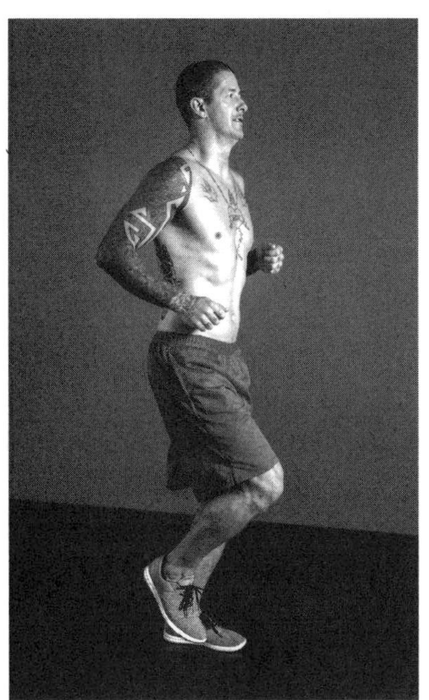

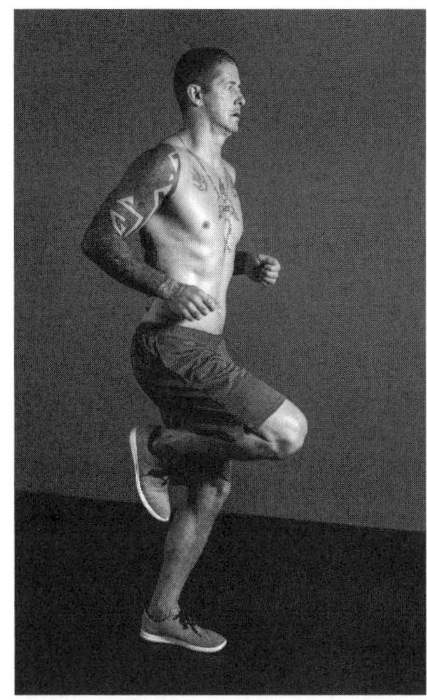

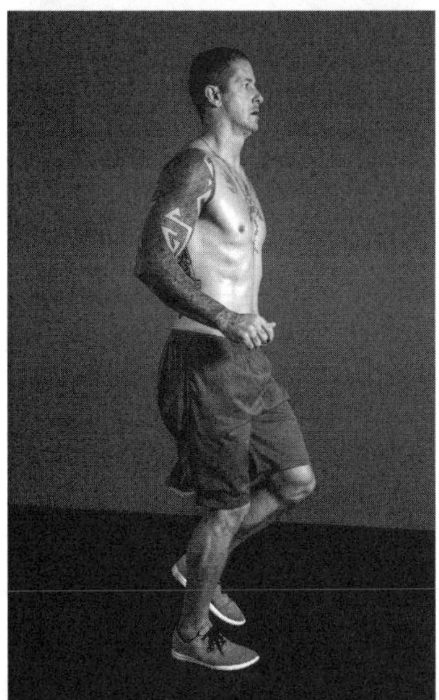

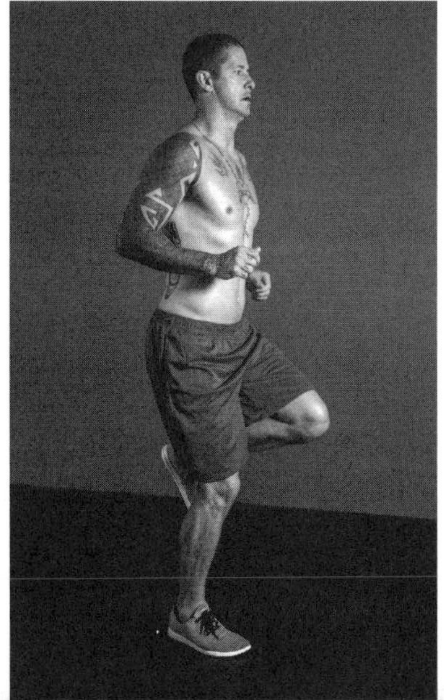

Exercises

BODY-WEIGHT EXERCISES

Air Squat

The air squat is one of the best body-weight exercises for improving hip and trunk strength; mastering this exercise will accelerate your skill improvement with other strength and conditioning exercises. Good form is crucial.

Start in a standing position, engaging your core muscles. Keep your back flat as you drive your hips back, push your arms out, and lower your trunk. Do not allow your knees to float out over your feet—this puts excessive pressure on the knees. Instead, keep shins vertical throughout the movement. Now drive your knees outward and keep your weight on your heels as you lower your hips. Don't let your heels come off the ground. Aim for 20 repetitions.

SCALE: Slow down and squat as deeply as your mobility currently allows, fighting for depth on each rep. Quality form is your number-one priority.

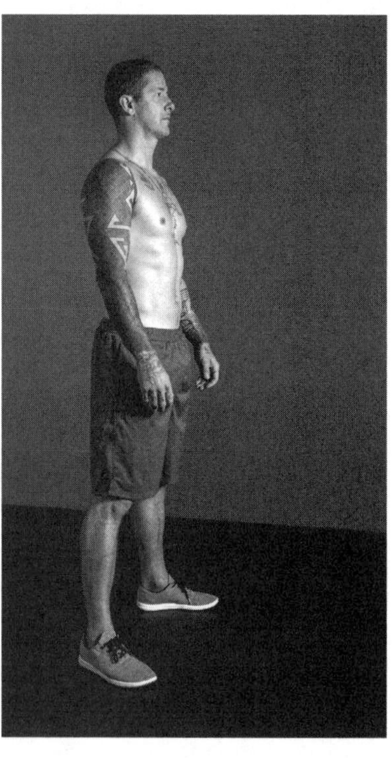

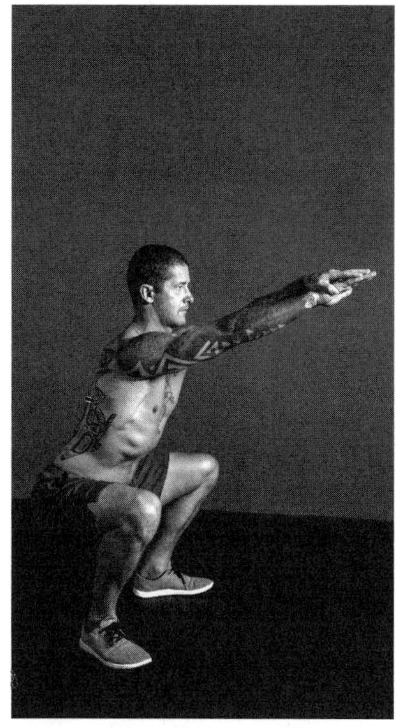

Pull-up

Engage your core and reach up for the pull-up bar. Use your back muscles to draw yourself upward. Clear the bar with your chin, and return.

SCALE: If you lack the upper-body strength to do dead-hang pull-ups, perform jumping pull-ups, jumping from the ground or a box to develop momentum to get you up over the bar. Another way to build strength is to slowly return to the start position of the pull-up to emphasize the negative pattern and build power. A workout partner can help by cupping your feet and giving you a lift.

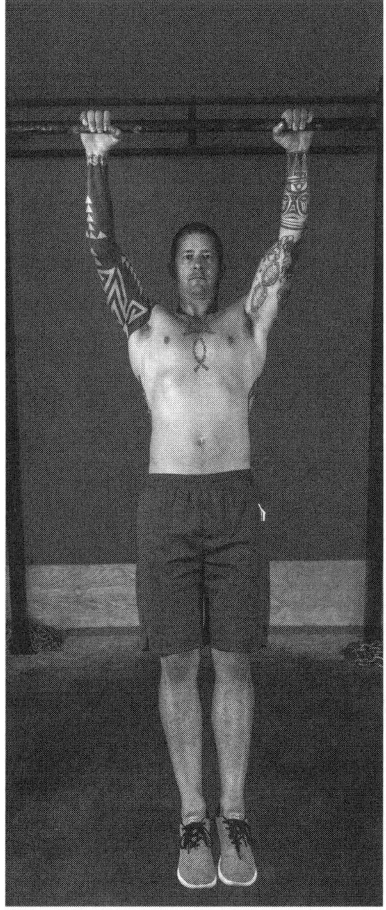

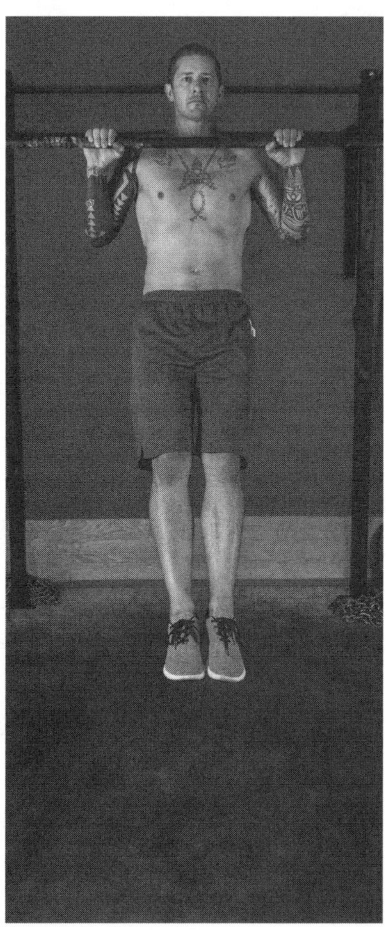

Ring Row

Where available, use a set of gymnastics rings and lower them to a few feet above the ground. Lie under the rings, facing up toward them. With the trunk engaged (as always), pull yourself up from the ground and draw your chest to the rings.

NOTE: This is also a scaling option for pull-ups.

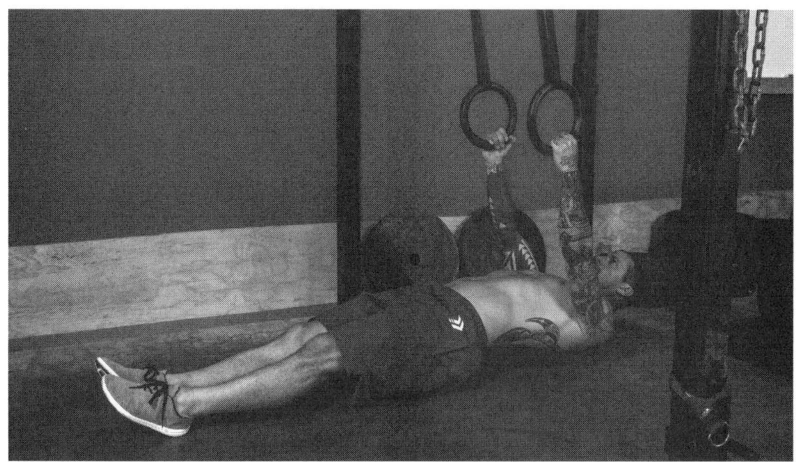

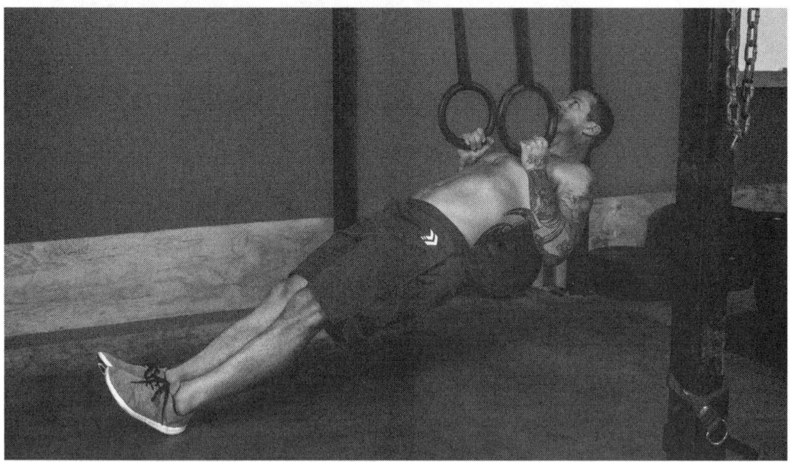

Push-up

Push-ups are an excellent pressing exercise and a great functional exercise that will do wonders for trunk strength and running form.

Start in a plank position with arms extended and elbows locked. Make sure your core is engaged, then lower your body so that your chest touches the ground. Keep elbows close to your body throughout and concentrate on channeling power from your trunk into the movement as you press upward for 1 rep.

SCALE: Reduce the length and intensity of your plank by dropping down to your knees.

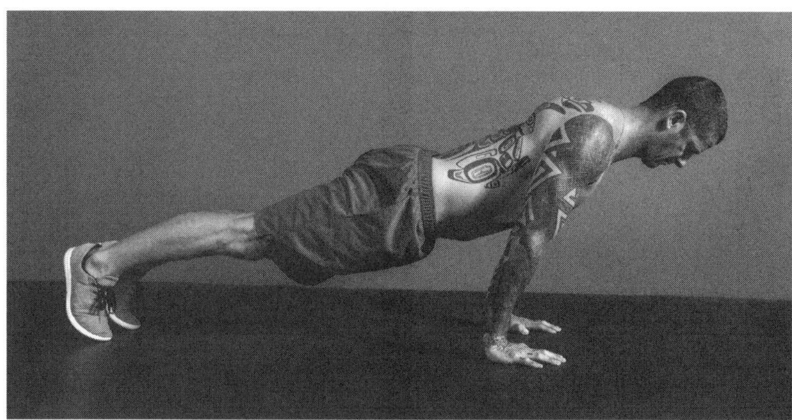

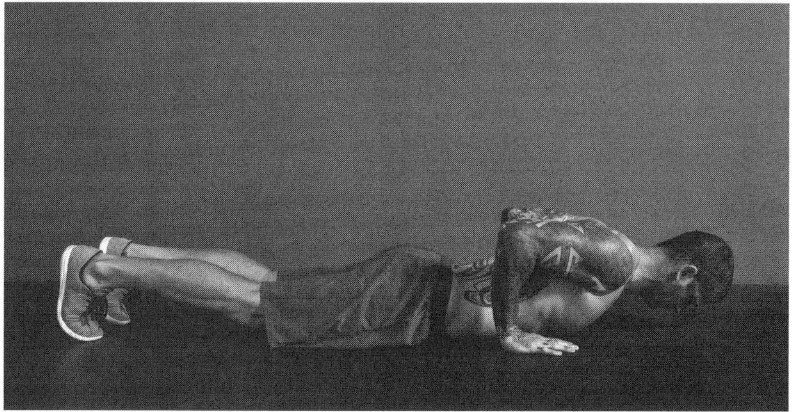

Sit-up

Start with your legs bent and feet flat on the ground and use your core to pull your upper body into an upright position. Return and repeat.

SCALE: Have a workout partner hold your ankles, which will allow you to engage your hip flexors and legs to assist in the exercise.

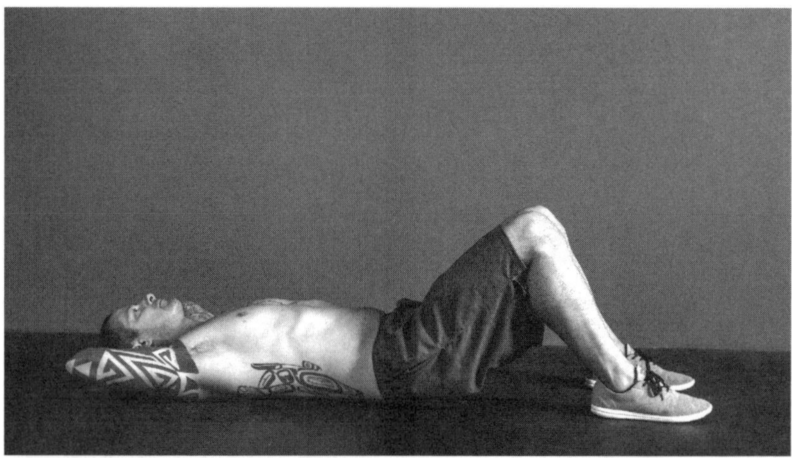

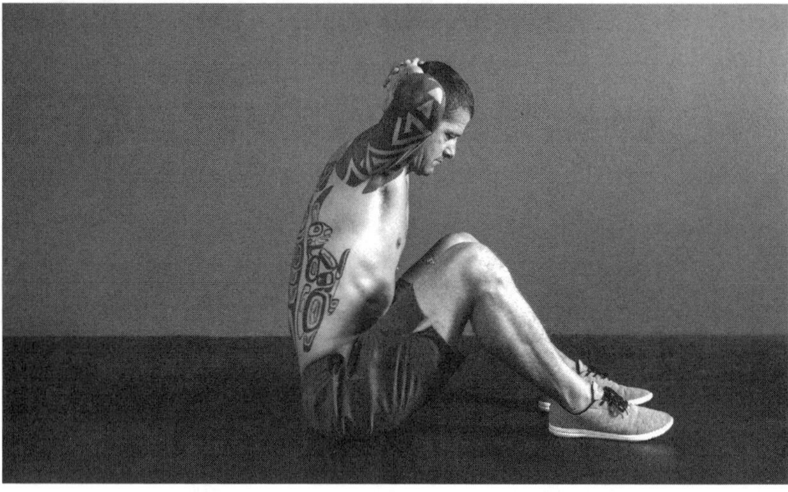

V-up

This great trunk exercise will help you with your hollow rock drill and running form.

Start flat on the ground with your arms stretched out overhead. Draw your legs and arms upward and together on their way to a meeting in the middle. Return and repeat.

SCALE: Alternate crunches with leg raises until you can combine them into one smooth movement.

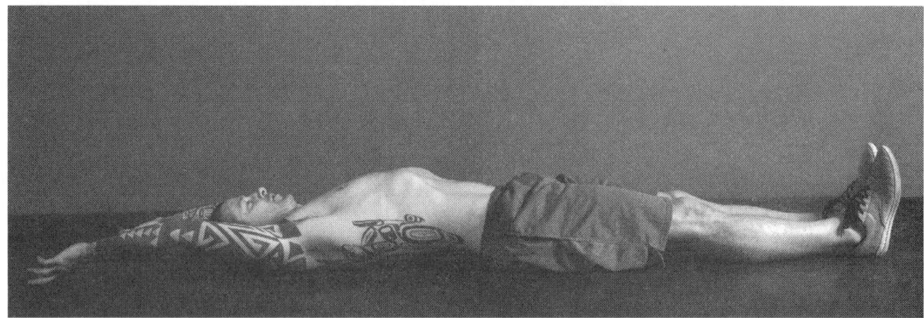

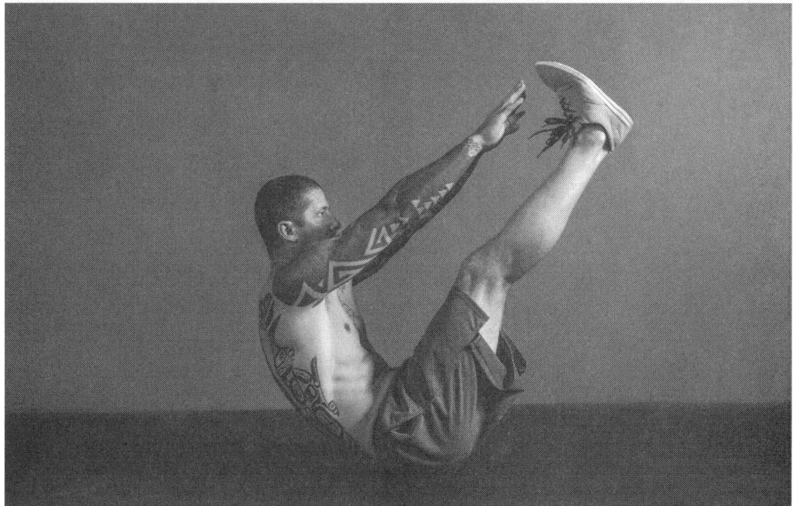

Toes-to-Bar

Hanging from a bar, use your core strength to draw your toes up to your hands, then return to the dead hang for 1 rep.

SCALE: Draw your knees to your elbows.

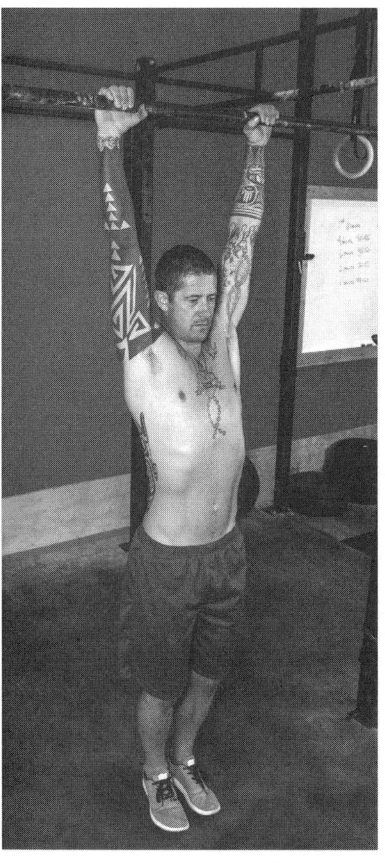

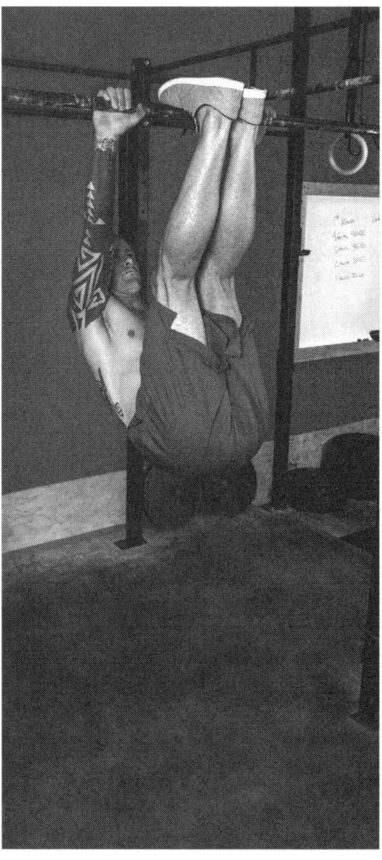

Burpee

This classic functional movement exercise creates a high metabolic demand and is loved and hated by football players and soldiers everywhere.

Start in a standing position, with core engaged, and drop facedown with hands on the ground. Kick out into a push-up position, maintaining an engaged core, and perform a push-up with elbows close to the body and retaining a 45-degree angle. Pull your feet back beneath you as you stand and clap overhead.

SCALE: The primary obstacle of the burpee is the metabolic demand. Pace yourself to build up stamina.

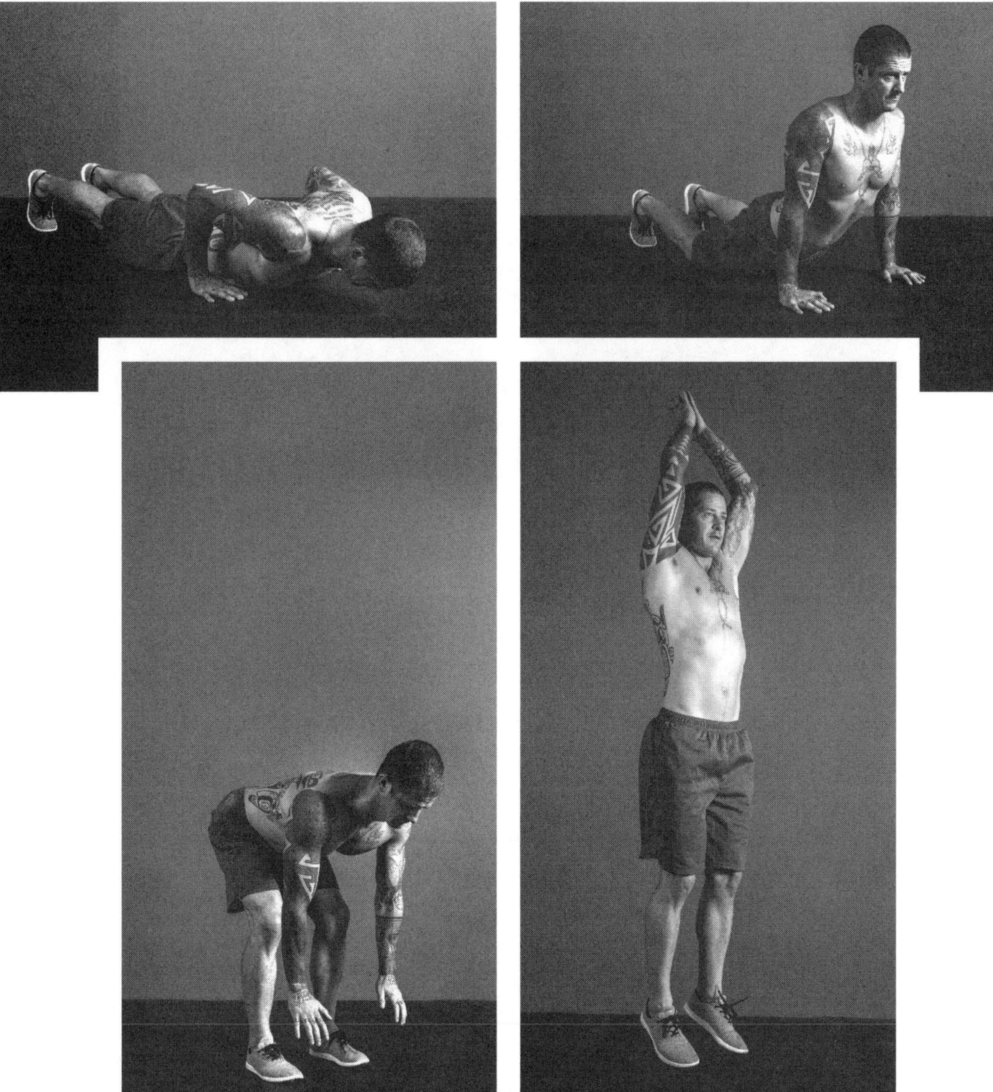

Box Step-up

Use a 16- or 20-inch box. Face the box, engage your core, and step up onto the box. Make sure your foot remains neutral throughout—don't allow it to spin outward, ducklike. Use your hips to drive yourself up on top of the box, and return.

SCALE: Start with a lower box and work your way up.

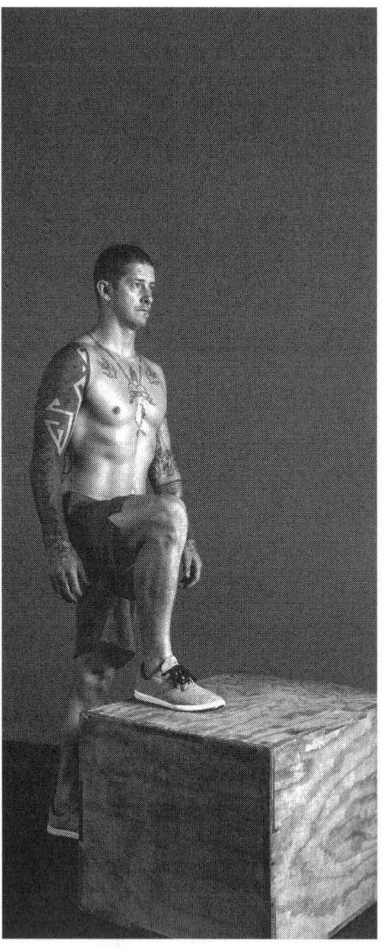

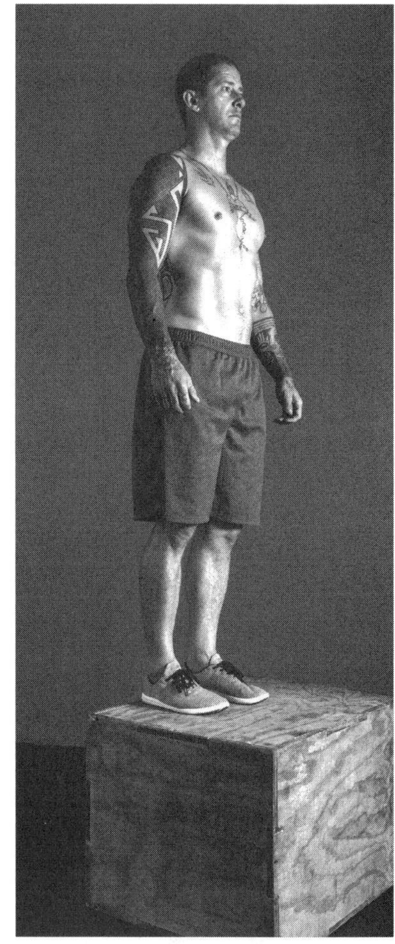

Lunge

Throughout the exercise, focus on engaging your core, hips, and hamstrings. Keep your shins and torso as vertical as possible.

From a standing position, take a long step forward and drop downward—using your hips to control the movement—and touch the opposite knee to the ground. Now power your body upward with your trunk muscles, returning to a standing position. Repeat on the other side.

SCALE: Drop your knee down as far as you are able, even if you cannot touch the ground, and work toward achieving the full range of motion required.

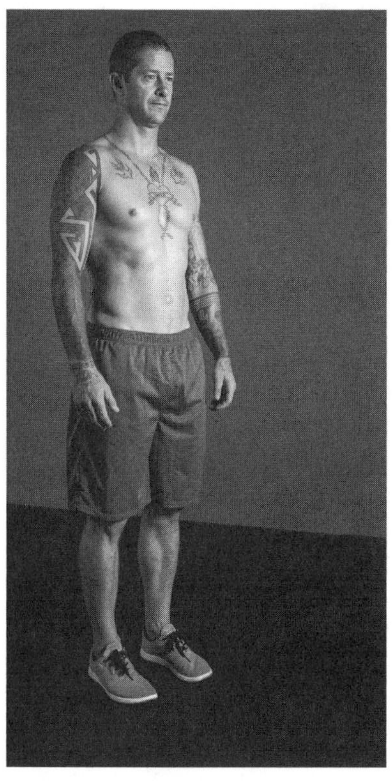

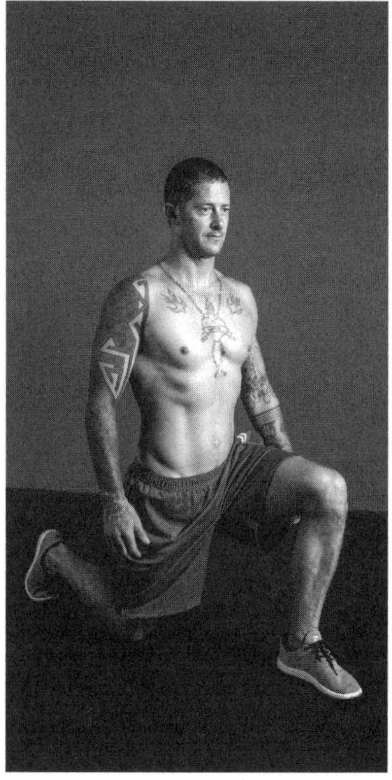

EXERCISES

Dip

This is a great body-weight exercise for strengthening arms, shoulders, and core stabilizing muscles.

Grip a pair of gymnastic rings and engage your core. Aim to engage core muscles as you press upward until elbows are locked. Keep your elbows in throughout, and avoid leaning forward. Lower your body so that your chest is even with the rings for a count of 1. Repeat.

SCALE: Use parallel bars instead of rings. Additional scaling can be achieved by looping a band from your grip to beneath your knees.

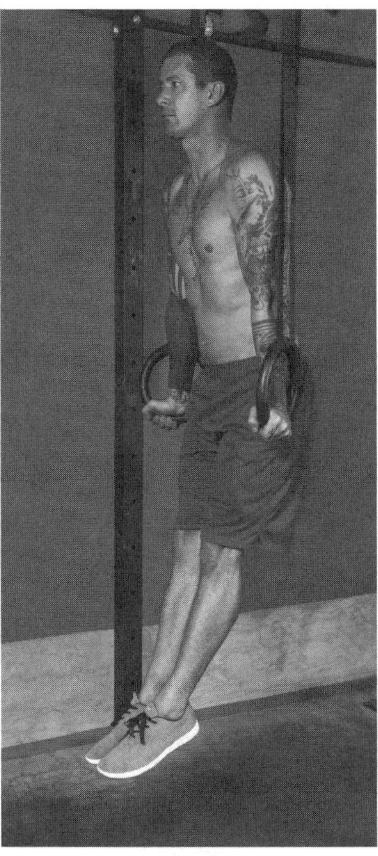

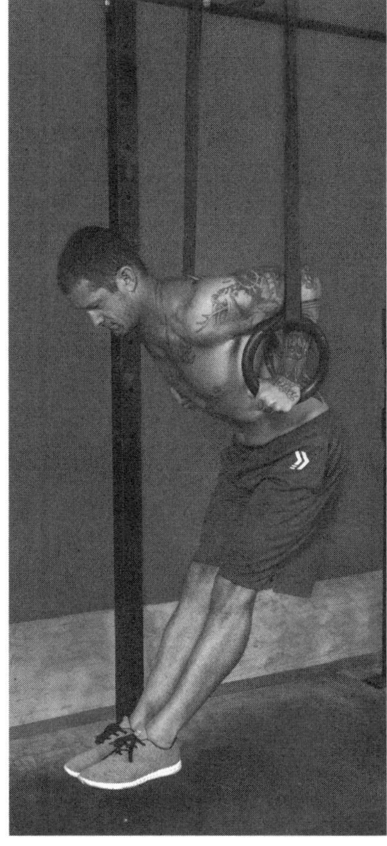

Double Under

In this jump-rope exercise, the rope passes below you twice in a single jump. It requires rhythm and takes practice to master, but jumping rope is a terrific exercise to aid you in your quest for good running form and is also great for strengthening your feet and ankles. Engage your core and work on developing a quick movement of the wrists.

SCALE: Practice single rope passes until you gain enough skill and strength to double up.

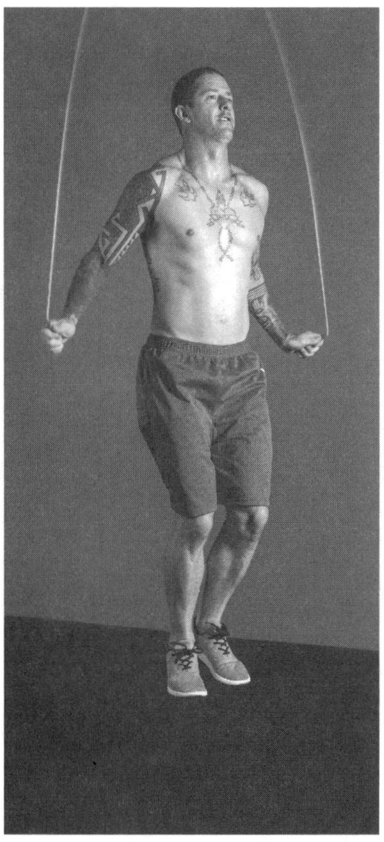

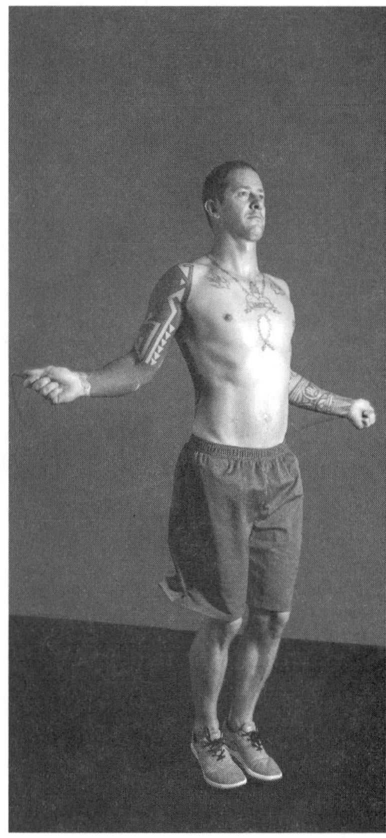

Exercises Using Weights

FARMER'S WALK

This is an excellent trunk-strengthening exercise.

Start by lifting a dumbbell or kettlebell in each hand, and then begin walking a predetermined distance, typically 10 to 20 yards. Repeat.

SCALE: Use lighter weights or shorten the walking distance.

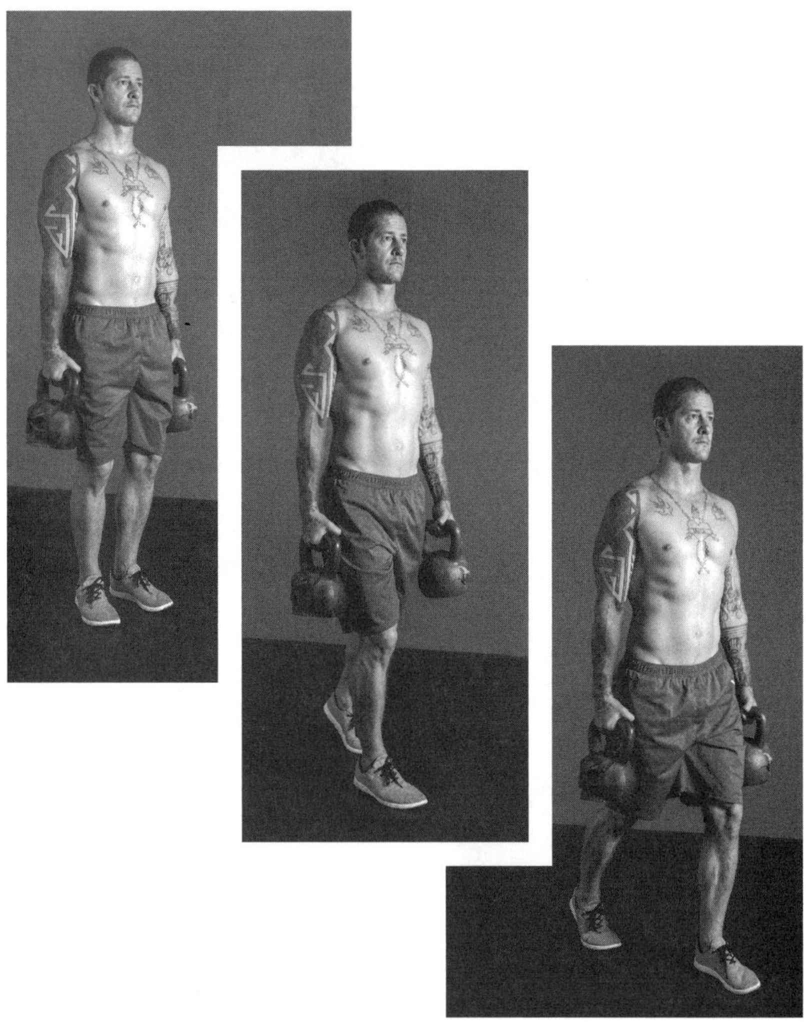

Back Squat

The back squat is a loaded version of the air squat, with a barbell placed across your shoulders and an appropriate weight load. The keys of the back squat are initiating the movement with your hamstrings, keeping your shins vertical and core engaged, and pressing your knees outward until your hip crease breaks the plane of your knees. Drive upward to a fully standing position for 1 rep.

SCALE: Stay with the unloaded air squat, or use a lightweight bar such as a PVC pipe.

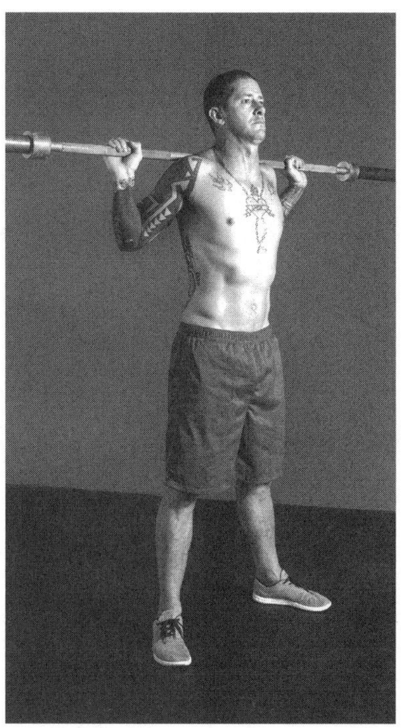

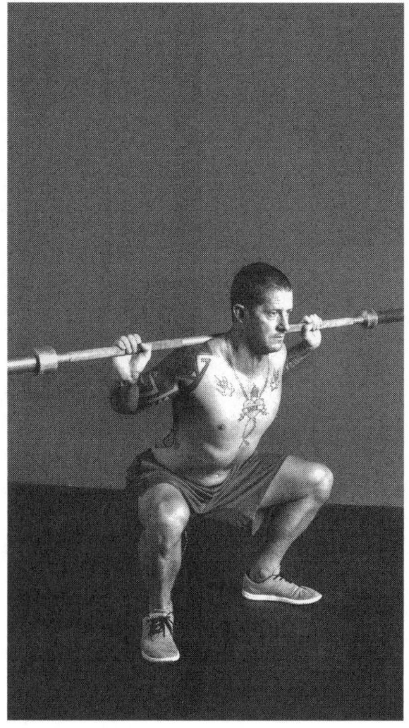

Kettlebell Swing

This exercise might seem at first to be an arm exercise, but when properly performed, it builds trunk strength and develops the flow of power from the large muscles of the hips through the extremities. The key is to engage your hips.

Start in a standing position with both hands on the kettlebell and feet shoulder width apart. Draw your hips back and allow the bell to swing beneath you; then, with a sharp snap of the hips, launch the kettlebell into an arc that rises to chest level or above the head. Allow gravity to bring the kettlebell back down to the starting position. Keep good posture and engage your core throughout the movement.

SCALE: Practice this movement with a lighter kettlebell at first, progressing in weight as your strength improves.

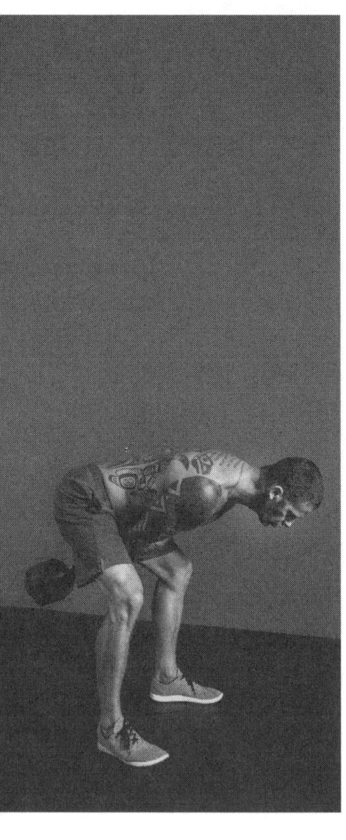

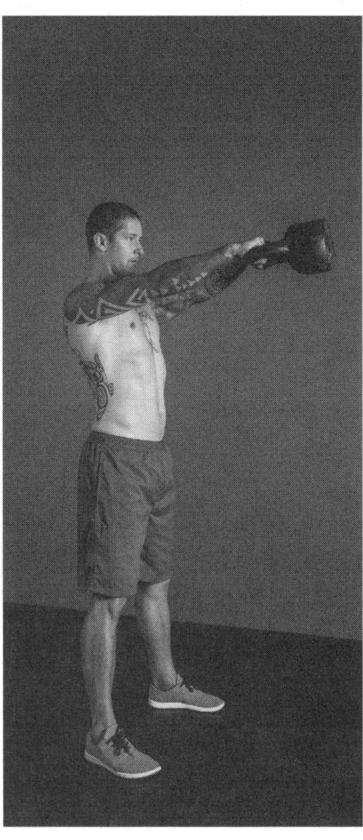

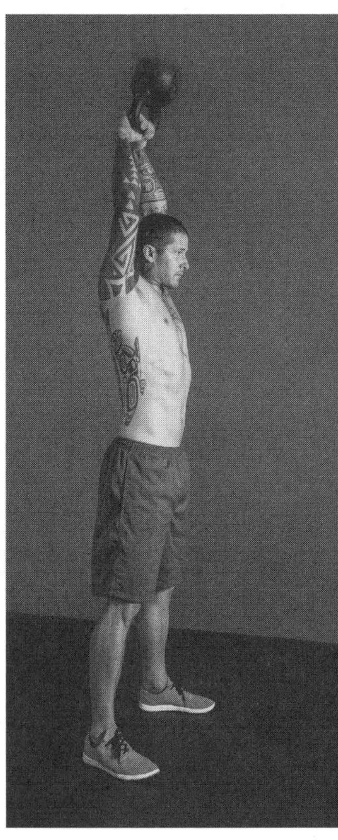

Deadlift

This is a classic lower-back and hip strengthening exercise.

Face a barbell, with your shins touching the bar, and engage your core as you lower your upper body, bending the knees slightly, and grip the bar with hands just outside shoulder width. Keep your back flat throughout the movement.

Begin the deadlift by engaging your hips and hamstrings as you drive your heels into the ground. Keep shins vertical as you fully extend your trunk. The path of the bar should follow a line that is close to the body throughout the lift. Focus on your hips as you drive your trunk backward and lower the bar to the ground, using the same bar path that you followed in the extension part of the lift.

SCALE: Practice the deadlift with a PVC pipe or unloaded barbell to get the movement down, then begin adding weight. Note that an Olympic-style bar by itself weighs 45 pounds.

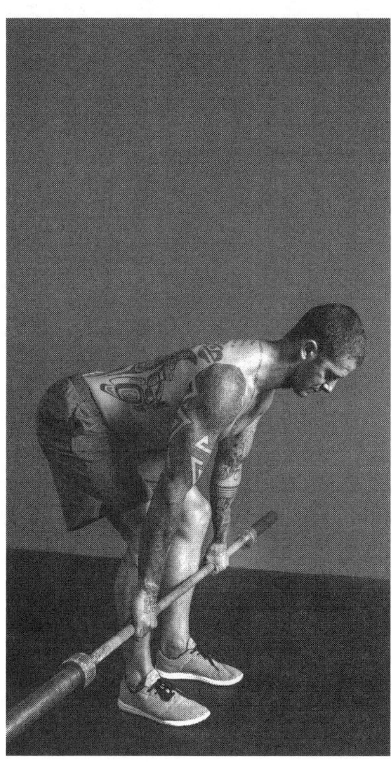

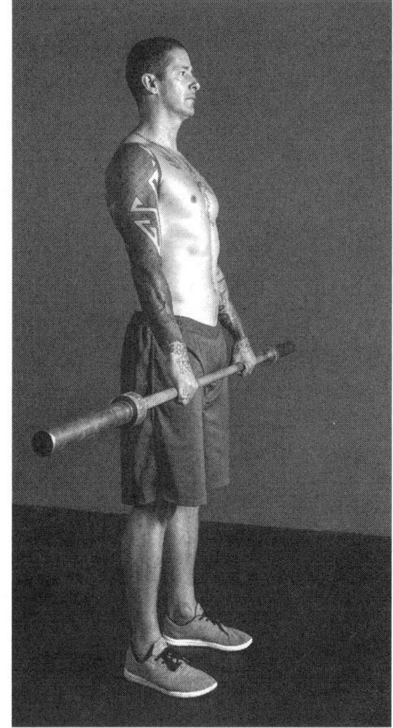

Front Squat

Place the barbell on the front of your shoulders and across your chest. With the weight racked in front of your body, you'll engage more of the quads than you do in an air squat. Throughout the front squat, concentrate on driving with the hips and powering upward with your elbows.

SCALE: Use a PVC pipe or unloaded barbell.

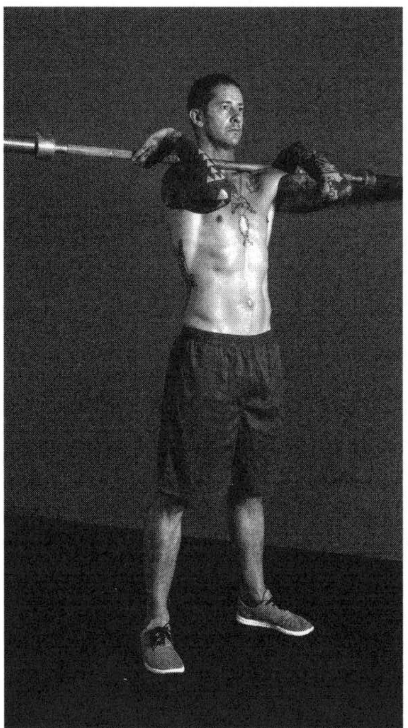

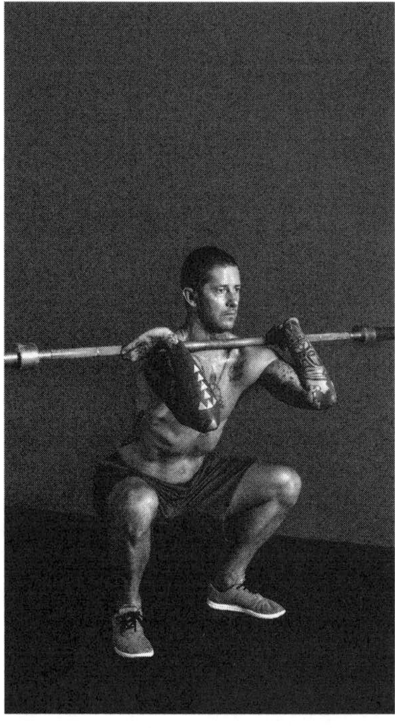

Standing Press

The basic standing press is a pure strength move.

Raise a barbell to shoulder height. Engage your trunk and place your hands on the bar, just outside your shoulders, with your feet directly beneath your hips. Drive the bar upward until it is overhead and your arms are fully locked out, then return until the bar is racked on the front of your shoulders and repeat.

SCALE: Practice this movement with a bar only until you have mastered the movement and have developed enough strength to add additional weight. Note that an Olympic-style bar by itself weighs 45 pounds.

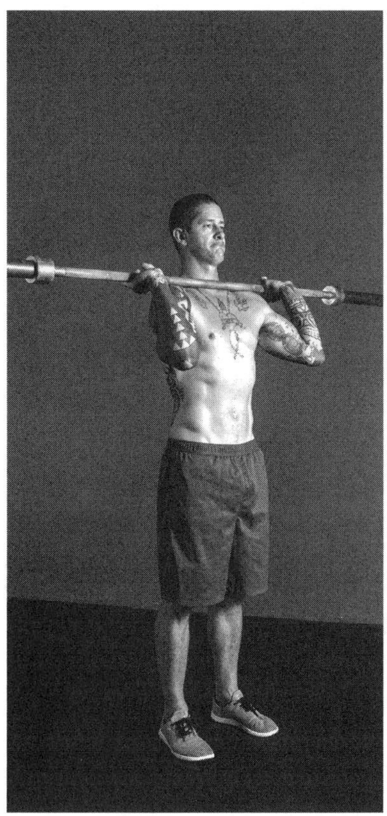

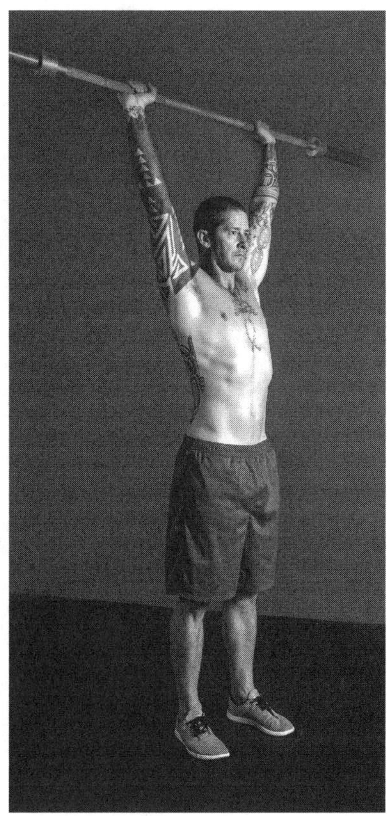

EXERCISES

Wall Ball

This exercise is a metabolic firestorm that develops mobility, coordination, and stamina.

Place your hands underneath a medicine ball and center it beneath your chin and against your chest. Drop down as if performing a front squat, with your hip crease passing beneath the plane of your knees, then explode upward, powering the ball with the momentum generated by your trunk. After full extension, press the ball into the air, shooting for a mark on a building or wall, 10 feet above the ground. Catch the ball on the rebound and retrace the same pathway back to the bottom of the squat for 1 rep. Repeat.

SCALE: Start with a sports ball, such as a volleyball or kickball, and progress to a heavier medicine ball as your strength improves.

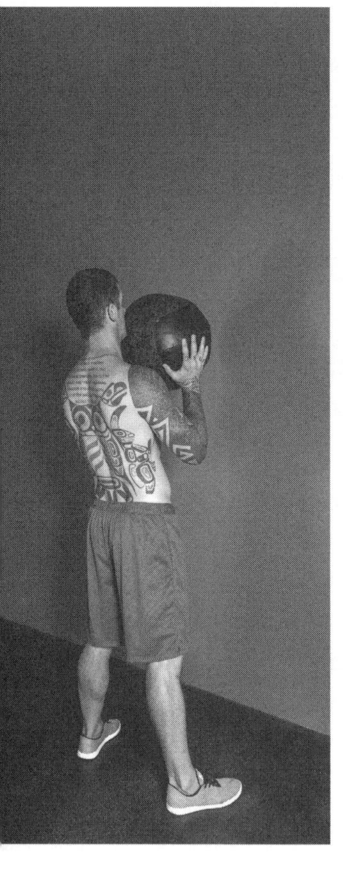

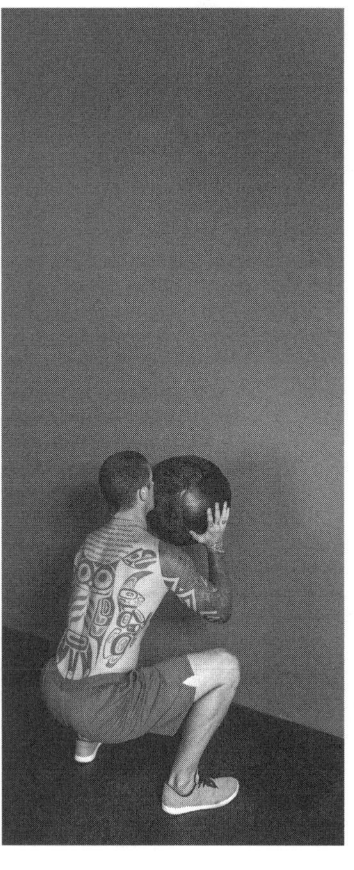

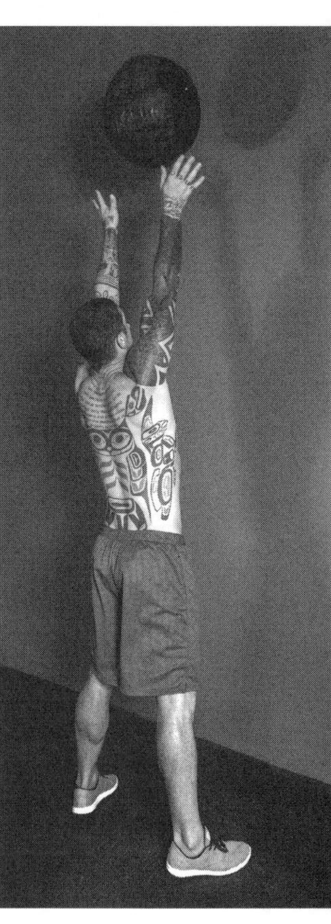

Push Press

The push press draws on more full-body power than a regular press.

With the bar racked on the front of your shoulders, perform a "dip and drive" by bending at the knees and drawing up power in the hips. Then quickly explode upward (as in the wall ball exercise) so that the energy you created from the dip and drive pushes the bar into the air as you press it into full extension—knees and elbows locked.

As you develop this skill, you'll be able to push press considerably more weight than you can press.

SCALE: Practice the movement with a PVC pipe or unloaded bar, and slowly work up to adding weight.

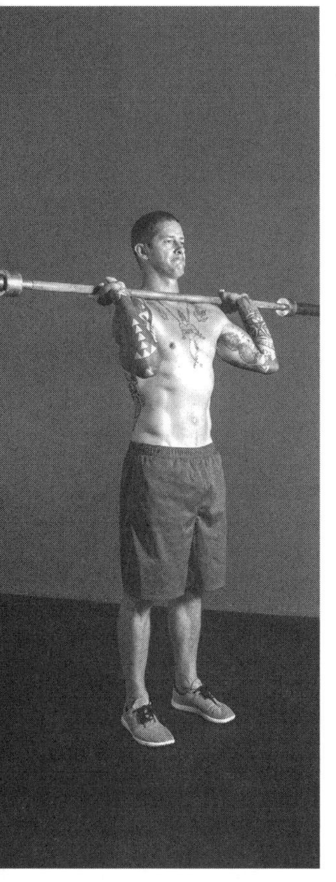

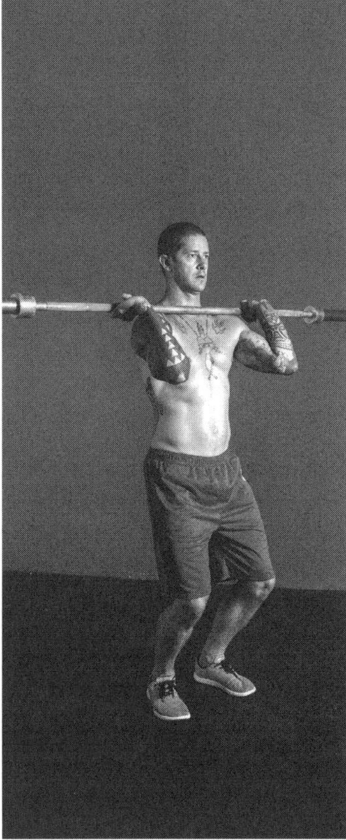

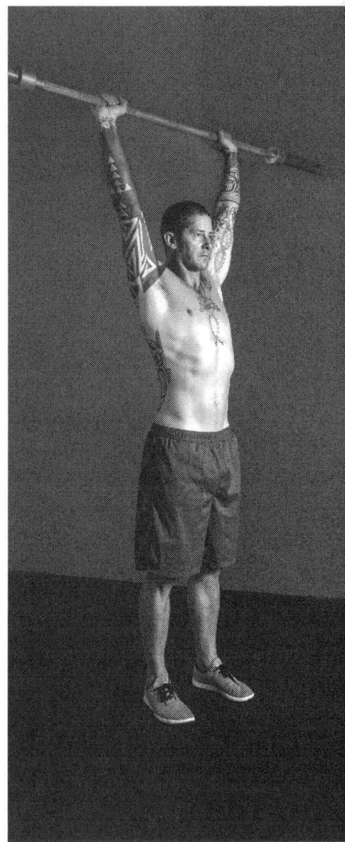

6-Week CFE Transition Programs

Tables 5.1 and 5.2 are two different 6-week CFE on-ramp schedules that introduce the method and prepare athletes for the race-specific training plans in Chapter 6. What lies at the heart of both of these programs is a core transition into a *skill-based* approach to running. In the course of 6 weeks, you will steadily build a new foundation of movement by incrementally adding training in running technique, cadence, and strength.

The first plan is designed for traditional runners who do not have any experience with CrossFit or other high-intensity strength and conditioning programs. It provides exposure to CrossFit through an emphasis on body-weight-based strength movements, such as push-ups and sit-ups, formulated in brief, CrossFit-style sessions.

Most CrossFit gyms offer on-ramp programs, but if you don't have access to such a program or prefer to work on your own, this 6-week plan is designed to be an accessible introduction. It requires no specialized equipment and can be easily followed in your home.

The second plan is designed for those with at least some CrossFit experience. Because these athletes already have a strength and conditioning base, their program begins with standard CrossFit workouts as part of the 6-week on-ramp program.

At first glance, the workouts in these programs might appear to be written in code, but in reality, they are easy to follow. Let's go through the structure of a skill session and demonstrate how it plays out. For example, on the first Tuesday of the Body-Weight Introduction to CrossFit and Running schedule, your workout is as follows:

3 drills + run 20 m betw. each

2 × (4 × :30 @ 94–96 cadence/rest 1:00 + 2:00 @ 91 cadence/rest 2:00)

10 × 50 m run barefoot in sand/grass, walk 50 m

This is what it means:

- After warming up, perform three drills from the drill section, with 20 meters of running between each drill repeat. (For example, start with hop with forward lean, run 20 meters, do the pulling wall drill, run another 20 meters, and finish with the alternating foot drill.)
- Next, perform four 30-second runs with an emphasis on cadence. Using a portable metronome set at 94 beeps per minute, time each pull of your left foot with the beep. Rest 1 minute after each run. Then do the whole set a second time.
- Next, run a longer distance at a slightly slower cadence. Set the metronome for 91 beeps per minute and run for 2 minutes, pulling your left foot in sync with the beat. Rest 2 minutes; then repeat the four 30-second runs and the 2-minute run.
- Finally, it's time for barefoot strength work. Run 50 meters in sand or grass at a comfortable pace while focusing on maintaining good mechanics and a fast cadence. Walk back to the starting line after each repetition. Perform this routine 10 times.

After cracking the workout code, you will be able to understand any of the notations contained in these schedules.

In both schedules, you will find key running skill sessions on Tuesdays, on Thursdays, and occasionally on weekends. Here you'll find drills, cadence work, and barefoot exercises, which together help build good running mechanics and high cadence.

Time spent exercising barefoot on the grass or in the sand will also build strength and elasticity into your feet. Along with jumping rope, simply spending time being barefoot will do wonders to strengthen the arch and the ankle complex. Short, consistent exposures over time will stress the foot in a way that is safe and extremely effective at restoring functionality and range of motion to the muscles and connective tissues, including the length of the heel cord.

If any exercise in either program feels out of reach, scale back the movement to something you can safely perform. A good way to do this is to reduce the intensity of the exercise by lowering the resistance or else dropping down the number of reps or the amount

TABLE 5.1: Body-Weight Introduction to CrossFit and Running

	M	T	W	
WEEK 1	**3 rounds NFT:** 5 pull-ups 10 push-ups 20 sit-ups	3 drills + run 20 m betw. each 2 × (4 × :30 @ 94–96 cadence/ rest 1:00 + 2:00 @ 91 cadence/ rest 2:00) 10 × 50 m run barefoot in sand/grass, walk 50 m	**3 rounds NFT:** 5 pull-ups 10 push-ups 15 lunges 20 sit-ups	
WEEK 2	**4 rounds FT:** 5 pull-ups 15 lunges 20 sit-ups	3 drills + run 20 m betw. each 2 × (4 × :30 @ 96–98 cadence/ rest 1:00 + 2:00 @ 92 cadence/ rest 2:00) 10 × 100 m run barefoot in sand/grass, walk 50 m	**4 rounds FT:** 5 pull-ups 10 push-ups 15 squats 20 sit-ups	

of time for which each exercise is to be repeated. For example, a recommended substitution for a pull-up is the supine ring row (see page 96): Using a pair of gymnastics rings lowered to near the floor, lie on your back and pull yourself up for a count of 1. Similarly, you can perform push-ups from your knees instead of from your toes.

You can also moderate the intensity of an exercise by breaking it up into two or more segments. For example, instead of 1 set of 100 sit-ups, you might do 4 sets of 25.

Once you have completed this program, you will be ready to design your own program using the plans in Chapter 6.

	T	F	S	S
	3 drills + run 20 m betw. each 2 × (4 × :30 @ 94–96 cadence/ rest 1:00 + 2:00 @ 91 cadence/ rest 2:00) 10 × 50 m run barefoot in sand/grass, walk 50 m	**5 rounds NFT:** 5 pull-ups 10 push-ups 20 sit-ups	**OPTIONAL:** 3 drills + run 20 m betw. each 2 × (4 × :30 @ 94–96 cadence/rest 1:00 + 2:00 @ 91 cadence/ rest 2:00) 10 × 50 m run barefoot in sand/grass, walk 50 m	**OFF**
	3 drills + run 20 m betw. each 2 × (4 × :30 @ 96–98 cadence/ rest 1:00 + 2:00 @ 92 cadence/ rest 2:00) 10 × 100 m run barefoot in sand/grass, walk 50 m	**5 rounds FT:** 5 pull-ups 10 push-ups 15 lunges 20 sit-ups	**OPTIONAL:** 3 drills + run 20 m betw. each 2 × (4 × :30 @ 96–98 cadence/ rest 1:00 + 2:00 @ 92 cadence/rest 2:00) 10 × 100 m run barefoot in sand/grass, walk 50 m	**OFF**

CONTINUED

CONTINUED

TABLE 5.1: Body-Weight Introduction to CrossFit and Running

	M	T	W	
WEEK 3	**10 min. AMRAP:** 5 pull-ups 15 air squats 20 sit-ups	3 drills + run 20 m betw. each 2 × (4 × :45 @ 98–100 cadence/ rest 1:30 + 2 drills + 3:00 @ 94 cadence/ rest 2:00) 10 × 100 m run barefoot in sand/grass, walk 100 m	**1 round FT:** 25 pull-ups 50 push-ups 75 lunges 100 sit-ups, then 2 min. hollow rock work	
WEEK 4	**1 round FT:** 50 push-ups 75 lunges 100 sit-ups	3 drills + run 20 m betw. each 2 × (4 × 1:00 @ 98–100 cadence/ rest 1:30 + 2 drills + 4:00 @ 94 cadence/ rest 2:00) 10 × 100 m run barefoot in sand/grass, walk 100 m	**10 rounds NFT:** 5 pull-ups 10 push-ups 15 air squats 20 sit-ups	
WEEK 5	**1 round FT:** 35 pull-ups 65 push-ups 90 lunges 115 sit-ups	3 drills + run 20 m betw. each 2 × (4 × 1:00 @ 100 + cadence/ rest 1:30 + 2 drills + 4:00 @ 95 cadence/ rest 2:00) 10 × 100 m run barefoot in sand/grass, walk 100 m	**15 min. AMRAP:** 5 pull-ups 10 push-ups 15 air squats 20 sit-ups	
WEEK 6	**1 round FT:** 50 pull-ups 75 push-ups 100 squats 125 sit-ups	3 drills + run 20 m betw. each 2 × (4 × 1:30 @ 100+ cadence/ rest 1:30 + 2 drills + 6:00 @ 95 cadence/ rest 2:00) 10 × 100 m run barefoot in sand/grass, walk 100 m	**4 rounds NFT:** 25 pull-ups 25 push-ups 25 lunges 25 sit-ups	

	T	F	S	S
	3 drills + run 20 m betw. each 2 × (4 × :45 @ 98–100 cadence/ rest 1:30 + 2 drills + 3:00 @ 94 cadence/ rest 2:00) 10 × 100 m run barefoot in sand/grass, walk 100 m	**5 rounds FT:** 5 pull-ups 10 push-ups 15 lunges 20 sit-ups, then 2 min. hollow rock work	**OPTIONAL:** 3 drills + run 20 m betw. each 2 × (4 × :45 @ 98-100 cadence/ rest 1:30 + 2 drills + 3:00 @ 94 cadence/rest 2:00) 10 × 100 m run barefoot in sand/grass, walk 100 m	**OFF**
	3 drills + run 20 m betw. each 2 × (4 × 1:00 @ 98–100 cadence/ rest 1:30 + 2 drills + 4:00 @ 94 cadence/ rest 2:00) 10 × 100 m run barefoot in sand/grass, walk 100 m	**10 min. AMRAP:** 5 pull-ups 10 push-ups 15 air squats	**OPTIONAL:** 3 drills + run 20 m betw. each 2 × (4 × 1:00 @ 98–100 cadence/ rest 1:30 + 2 drills + 4:00 @ 94 cadence/rest 2:00) 10 × 100 m run barefoot in sand/grass, walk 100 m	**OFF**
	3 drills + run 20 m betw. each 2 × (4 × 1:00 @ 100+ cadence/ rest 1:30 + 2 drills + 4:00 @ 95 cadence/ rest 2:00) 10 × 100 m run barefoot in sand/grass, walk 100 m	**5 rounds FT:** 5 pull-ups 10 push-ups 15 lunges 20 sit-ups	**OPTIONAL:** 3 drills + run 20 m betw. each 2 × (4 × 1:00 @ 100+ cadence/ rest 1:30 + 2 drills + 4:00 @ 95 cadence/rest 2:00) 10 × 100 m run barefoot in sand/grass, walk 100 m	OFF
	3 drills + run 20 m betw. each 2 × (4 × 1:30 @ 100+ cadence/ rest 1:30 + 2 drills + 6:00 @ 95 cadence/ rest 2:00) 10 × 100 m run barefoot in sand/grass, walk 100 m	**20 min. AMRAP:** 5 pull-ups 10 push-ups 15 air squats	**OPTIONAL:** 3 drills + run 20 m betw. each 2 × (4 × 1:30 @ 100+ cadence/ rest 1:30 + 2 drills + 6:00 @ 95 cadence/rest 2:00) 10 × 100 m run barefoot in sand/grass, walk 100 m	OFF

TABLE 5.2: Introduction to Running for Established CrossFitters

	M	T	W	T	
WEEK 1	CrossFit	3 drills + run 20 m betw. each 2 × (4 × :30 @ 94–96 cadence/ 1:00 rest + 2:00 @ 91 cadence/ 2:00 rest) 10 × 50 m run barefoot in sand/grass, walk 50 m	CrossFit (run bias) or OFF	3 drills + run 20 m betw. each 2 × (4 × :30 @ 94–96 cadence/ 1:00 rest + 2:00 @ 91 cadence/ 2:00 rest) 10 × 50 m run barefoot in sand/grass, walk 50 m	
WEEK 2	CrossFit	3 drills + run 20 m betw. each 2 × (4 × :30 @ 96–98 cadence/ 1:00 rest + 2:00 @ 92 cadence/ 2:00 rest) 10 × 100 m run barefoot in sand/grass, walk 50 m	CrossFit (run bias) or OFF	3 drills + run 20 m betw. each 2 × (4 × :30 @ 96–98 cadence/ 1:00 rest + 2:00 @ 92 cadence/ 2:00 rest) 10 × 100 m run barefoot in sand/grass, walk 50 m	
WEEK 3	CrossFit	3 drills + run 20 m betw. each 2 × (4 × :45 @ 98–100 cadence/ 1:30 rest + 2 drills + 3:00 @ 94 cadence/ 2:00 rest) 10 × 100 m run barefoot in sand/grass, walk 100 m	CrossFit	3 drills + run 20 m betw. each 2 × (4 × :45 @ 98–100 cadence/ 1:30 rest + 2 drills + 3:00 @ 94 cadence/ 2:00 rest) 10 × 100 m run barefoot in sand/grass, walk 100 m	
WEEK 4	CrossFit	3 drills + run 20 m betw. each 2 × (4 × 1:00 @ 98–100 cadence/ 1:30 rest + 2 drills + 4:00 @ 94 cadence/ 2:00 rest) 10 × 100 m run barefoot in sand/grass, walk 100 m	CrossFit or OFF	3 drills + run 20 m betw. each 2 × (4 × 1:00 @ 98–100 cadence/ 1:30 rest + 2 drills + 4:00 @ 94 cadence/ 2:00 rest) 10 × 100 m run barefoot in sand/grass, walk 100 m	

	F	S	S
	CrossFit or OFF	CrossFit or OFF	3 drills + run 20 m betw. each 2 × (4 × :30 @ 94–96 cadence/ 1:00 rest + 2:00 @ 91 cadence/ 2:00 rest) 10 × 50 m run barefoot in sand/grass, walk 50 m
	CrossFit or OFF	3 drills + run 20 m betw. each 2 × (4 × :30 @ 96–98 cadence/ 1:00 rest + 2:00 @ 92 cadence/ 2:00 rest) 10 × 100 m run barefoot in sand/grass, walk 50 m	CrossFit
	CrossFit or OFF	3 drills + run 20 m betw. each 2 × (4 × :45 @ 98–100 cadence/ 1:30 rest + 2 drills + 3:00 @ 94 cadence/ 2:00 rest) 10 × 100 m run barefoot in sand/grass, walk 100 m	CrossFit
	CrossFit (run bias) or OFF	CrossFit	3 drills + run 20 m betw. each 2 × (4 × 1:00 @ 98–100 cadence/ 1:30 rest + 2 drills + 4:00 @ 94 cadence/ 2:00 rest) 10 × 100 m run barefoot in sand/grass, walk 100 m

CONTINUED

CONTINUED

TABLE 5.2: Introduction to Running for Established CrossFitters

	M	T	W	T	
WEEK 5	CrossFit	3 drills + run 20 m betw. each 2 × (4 × 1:00 @ 100+ cadence/ 1:30 rest + 2 drills + 4:00 @ 95 cadence/ 2:00 rest) 10 × 100 m run barefoot in sand/grass, walk 100 m	CrossFit or OFF	3 drills + run 20 m betw. each 2 × (4 × 1:00 @ 100+ cadence/ 1:30 rest + 2 drills + 4:00 @ 95 cadence/ 2:00 rest) 10 × 100 m run barefoot in sand/grass, walk 100 m	
WEEK 6	CrossFit	3 drills + run 20 m betw. each 2 × (4 × 1:30 @ 100+ cadence/ 1:30 rest + 2 drills + 6:00 @ 95 cadence/ 2:00 rest) 10 × 100 m run barefoot in sand/grass, walk 100 m	CrossFit	3 drills + run 20 m betw. each 2 × (4 × 1:30 @ 100+ cadence/ 1:30 rest + 2 drills + 6:00 @ 95 cadence/ 2:00 rest) 10 × 100 m run barefoot in sand/grass, walk 100 m	

CFE Workouts for Your Race-Specific Training Plans

Once you have mastered the 6-week transition program, you are ready to advance to the next CFE level. In Chapter 6, you will find full CFE training plans that are tailored for a range of specific race distance goals, from the 5K to the ultramarathon. These plans run from 8 to 12 weeks and guide you through all aspects of a CFE race-training plan.

Each of the training plans calls for several CrossFit strength workouts each week. You can decide exactly what you'll be doing in those workouts, or you can choose from the list of short CrossFit routines provided in this section. Each of these workouts can be

	F	S	S
	CrossFit or OFF	3 drills + run 20 m betw. each 2 × (4 × 1:00 @ 100+ cadence/ 1:30 rest + 2 drills + 4:00 @ 95 cadence/ 2:00 rest) 10 × 100 m run barefoot in sand/grass, walk 100 m	CrossFit
	CrossFit or OFF	CrossFit or OFF	3 drills + run 20 m betw. each 2 × (4 × 1:30 @ 100+ cadence/ 1:30 rest + 2 drills + 6:00 @ 95 cadence/ 2:00 rest) 10 × 100 m run barefoot in sand/grass, walk 100 m

plugged into your training plan whenever a CrossFit workout is called for.

Feel free to vary the CFE exercises that you choose, as well as the volume of your CFE workouts. This is your workout plan, and you get to decide what to do. The only rules are to ensure that you maintain a variety of movements and to be sure to include the drill work.

Each of these workouts can be performed in a basement, garage, or backyard or at a fitness facility. Alternatively, you can buy a day pass at your local CrossFit box facility. The policies for visiting a CrossFit gym for a single day vary from box to box, but you should be able to find all the necessary information on any box's web site.

As with the 6-week transition program, if you find yourself struggling to maintain proper form while performing any of these exercises, remember that you can scale back the movement or the number of rounds or the workout time to something you can accomplish.

Note that one group of CrossFit movements that is not included here consists of the primary Olympic lifting moves such as snatches, cleans, and split jerks. These are advanced movements that require exceptional mobility and can be dangerous if not performed correctly. For that reason, we recommend that you learn Olympic lifting basics under the supervision of a good coach.

If it is within your means to work with a coach, learning to perform Olympic lifts can be of great benefit because they require a wide range of athletic capacity. The snatch, for example, tests your ability to lift a large load of weight directly from the floor to over your head, with arms extended, in one swift, explosive movement. You might assume this movement is simply a matter of raw strength, but in fact a snatch requires tremendous amounts of speed, coordination, and mobility. Perhaps the most crucial benefit for runners in learning to perform an Olympic lift is that it teaches you how to channel the power of the hips outward to the limbs, transferring power through this kinetic chain.

Remember, though, that just about all compound movements provide some or all of the same benefits, often without the technical challenge of Olympic power lifting. Mastering a deep air squat, for example, also helps connect an athlete to the power within the hips and hamstrings. The kettlebell swing is a dynamic movement that is another good first step toward getting a feel for how the power flows in an Olympic lift. If you try to swing a kettlebell just with your arms, you'll burn out in no time. The key is to generate power from the hips.

Sample CrossFit Workouts

4 rounds for time (RFT):
6 deadlifts
12 knees to elbows or toes-to-bar

7 minutes as many rounds as possible (AMRAP):
1 push-ups
15 kettlebell swings

10 minutes AMRAP:
9 V-ups
12 kettlebell swings
15 push-ups

6 minutes AMRAP:
max pull-ups
10 air squats

4 RFT:
3 deadlifts
6 push-ups
9 air squats

5 RFT:
12 push presses
12 wall ball shots

FT:
100 wall ball shots

5 RFT:
8 kettlebell swings
10 box jumps
12 burpees

20 minutes AMRAP (run bias):
400-m run
15 sit-ups
25 air squats

6 minutes AMRAP (run bias):
10 air squats
15 V-ups
100-m run

4 RFT:
10 knees to elbows
20 kettlebell swings
30 double unders

10 minutes AMRAP:
10 pull-ups
10 standing presses

15 minutes AMRAP (run bias):
20 push-ups
20 sit-ups
200-m run

10 minutes AMRAP:
12 push presses
12 wall ball shots

FT:
50-40-30-20-10 double unders/sit-ups

FT:
400-m farmer's walk with heavy dumbbells, followed by 5 burpees each time you set down weights

20-minute AMRAP:
5 pull-ups
10 push-ups
15 air squats

FT:
- 12-15-21-15-12 box jumps, push-ups

5 RFT:
- 10 pull-ups
- 15 kettlebell swings
- 20 push-ups

12 minutes AMRAP:
- 12 dips
- 9 air squats
- 12 burpees

FT:
- 25 pull-ups
- 50 push-ups
- 75 lunges
- 100 sit-ups

3 RFT:
- 25 pull-ups
- 25 air squats
- 25 sit-ups

Recovery Within a CFE Training Plan

Training and racing take their toll on the body, and improvement comes when a good recovery plan is part of the program. This is especially true when an athlete is working at high intensity. Nothing in this program is written in stone; as we've discussed, the athlete should scale back the load or difficulty of the work as necessary and should also take recovery days as needed.

We have said it before, but it bears repeating: A traditional runner with little or no strength and conditioning background must be patient when starting out with a CFE program. Adapting to the intensity in both the running and the strength and conditioning work will take time.

Start out with one of the 6-week transition programs outlined in Tables 5.1 and 5.2. From there, CFE athletes can adopt one of the race-specific programs or simply include in their own plan a minimum of four CrossFit workouts per week chosen from the exercise options listed. From what we've seen, four weekly CFE workouts produce the best results, but each runner is different. If you're making progress with three or even two CrossFit workouts per week, there's no reason to argue with that approach.

The key is to carefully monitor how you are feeling and to sensibly plan your workouts and recovery around that. In the following section, you will find specific recommendations for recovery.

Strength and Conditioning Recovery Circuit (S & C Recovery)

From the moment you step across the finish line of a race, every choice you make affects the speed and depth of your recovery. Close on the heels of a race, we advise clean eating, taking in plenty of fluids, and performing a functional fitness workout. A "recovery workout" may seem like an oxymoron, but consider your needs upon finishing a hard race: You are very tight, your tissues are soaked with toxins, and you are probably feeling sore and beat-up. This is the perfect time for a CFE workout!

If you don't believe it, try out the following protocol as soon as you can get to the gym after one of your B-level races (perhaps the early afternoon following a morning race) to see for yourself if it works.

3 rounds, 10 to 12 reps per set:

Sit-ups. Use the basic form, page 98.

Superman back extensions. Lying prone on the ground, use your core to simultaneously raise your arms and legs for 1 rep.

Kettlebell swings. Use the basic form, page 108.

Push-ups. Use the classic push-up, page 97, with an emphasis on midline stability. Squeeze your butt and activate your glutes to support your body as a rigid plank.

Air squats. Use the basic form, page 94.

A full recovery plan also includes massage, which removes waste from the muscles and breaks up adhesions that form between muscle cells after hard exertion and can inhibit movement. Healthy eating and hydration are also important to replace lost nutrients, with an extra emphasis on protein to supply material to rebuild damaged muscle tissue.

Finally, rest after your races and workouts is required to give the body an opportunity to release growth hormone and complete the healing process. In the training plans in Chapter 6, you will find these workouts sprinkled in to help you recover during your training.

PRACTICALLY SPEAKING: THE ART AND PRACTICE OF CFE

By now, it should be clear that CFE is a flexible, user-friendly program. However, becoming a CFE athlete doesn't happen overnight; patience and consistency are required. No one understands this better than CFE coaches. To get an idea of how a coach might introduce a runner to CFE, I talked with Valerie Hunt, who is a top CFE coach and seminar instructor based in Austin, Texas. Hunt has been coaching for 20 years and now oversees BVM CrossFit in Austin.

How do you work with runners who are new to the CFE program?

The first thing I do is teach them the skill of running as well as CrossFit elements. I use video analysis so they can see their running, and I explain how they will become faster and more efficient, especially as they get stronger with CrossFit. I film some of their lifts as well so they can see their form and progression.

I start them with alternating sets of skill drills and short intervals so they are learning and running together. This way, they get used to including intervals in their training and continue to value the skill. The CrossFit is usually two days a week in the beginning, building up to four to six days as their strength progresses.

What insights do you have for those wanting to get the most out of CrossFit Endurance?

Optimal value from CFE is being able to handle the two-a-day workouts that include a CrossFit workout and also a CFE running interval workout. The ideal situation is to have runners spend 6 weeks in a skill progression program for both the running and the CrossFit, then spend the next 6 to 12 weeks following the CFE program for their race. If they can commit to a longer period, even better. I use video analysis a lot in the beginning so they can understand that

CONTINUED

CONTINUED

I am progressing their volume along with their skill. Also, spending 20 to 30 minutes on rotating drills and running as a warm-up, plus the interval portion, helps them not miss all of those long runs because they are still spending up to an hour on the track.

What sort of tweaks have you made to the baseline CFE program?

If runners at first cannot manage the two-a-days in their schedule, I have them alternate CrossFit and CFE days. Also, if they want to keep in one of their longer runs, that's OK with me as long as they make sure to get their intervals done and they continue to get faster. I also add extra hip/core body-weight exercises for them that they can do at home, especially if they cannot make the standard four to six CrossFit workouts per week. It's amazing how much of a speed increase I have seen just from the continuation of the skill progressions and adding the interval training.

What other advice do you have for runners starting CFE?

Recovery is important. We use the CFE strength and recovery protocol, or a body-weight alternative that works just as well. I like to call it "hip recovery." I have them make it a routine piece of their training, especially after every running workout or race.

I prepare them for races. I encourage performing race simulations or have them sign up for B races to prepare for their A race. We also make sure to include practicing nutrition in their runs, workouts of the day, and time trial workouts—the same protocol that they will be using for the race. I try to teach my runners to always eat like it is race week so they are always aware of what works for them.

I also suggest including mobility exercises for the feet, ankles, hips, and shoulders in every warm-up. Learn these from the beginning, and they simply become a part of your pre-run habits.

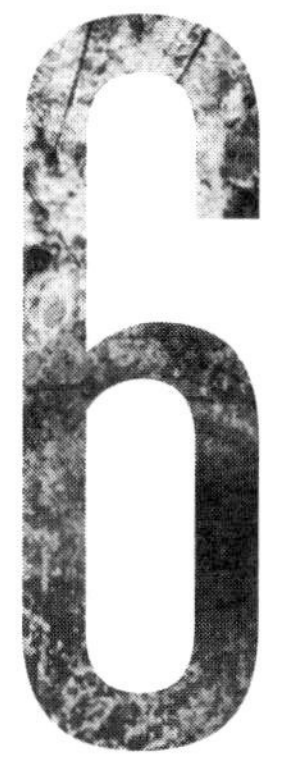

YOUR TRAINING PLANS

Why race? The need to be tested, perhaps; the need to take risks; and the chance to be number one.

—DR. GEORGE SHEEHAN, BEST-SELLING AUTHOR AND PHILOSOPHER

For many runners, training without having a race goal is like earning college credits without aiming to get your diploma. You might do it, but it can quickly seem pointless, and motivation tends to evaporate.

For many of us, racing is the glue that holds the whole program together. Having a race date circled on our calendar gets us out of bed in the morning and gets us on the roads and into the gym.

As I've explained, incorporating CrossFit Endurance into your program will make you more injury-resistant—or unbreakable, as in the title of this book. But, of course, that's not the only reason to do CFE. Improving form and strength, and staying *healthy*, will make you a better racer as well. To make the most of your training, however, you need to do more than just train with a race goal in mind; you should tailor your training plan to meet that race's specific demands. That's what this chapter is all about.

Every distance, from the 5K to an ultra, comes with its own unique set of opportunities and challenges. The first step to becoming a better racer is to recognize that you need a different plan for each race: different training distances, speeds, and race paces. If your race plans so far have mostly consisted of aiming to run the best you can, training and racing to specific pace goals can seem daunting. Don't let that faze you. Once your body fully learns the different gears at its disposal, you'll be able to match your training and racing strategies directly to the challenge that awaits you.

The training plans will prepare you for racing, but understanding *why* you're doing what you're doing is also crucial to your success. In the following pages, Brian MacKenzie offers an overview of how to use the CFE training plans and the CFE philosophy to accomplish your goals at specific race distances.

As you go through the plans, you should keep a few concepts in mind that apply throughout these workouts.

First, skill training is imperative. Don't blow it off. Skill work should not be skipped because it will ensure that you are not just running to build endurance but training to improve and maintain good form.

Second, you'll see how different cadences—that is, stride rate—are recommended for different workouts. Generally, Brian recommends a rapid cadence of up to 90 steps per foot per minute (or, more simply, 3 steps total per second). This ensures the maximum opportunity for applying force to generate speed while aligning the body to absorb impact most efficiently. The cadences that are specified for the different workouts here are a little higher than that; this will prepare your body to run at a cadence that can be easily sustained throughout a race and train you to be aware of even slight changes in cadence. During a race, this could mean the difference between a PR effort and hitting the wall. But don't let adherence to specific cadences distract you from the main task at hand in the workouts: to develop fast leg turnover while completing the assigned workout. In other words, coming close to perfect is perfect enough. The struggle to achieve the cadences is where the value is—it's the nature of how a new skill is built. To monitor your cadence, use a metronome or an app on your phone.

Third, be aware of deviations from the target split times for the speed workouts. An effective speed workout is hard but not as draining as a race. You should not be emptying your fuel tank during your workout. If you find that you are deviating by more than a second or two from one repeat to the next, you are slipping past training into racing and no longer training the body properly. The general idea is that you should be able to hold your pace or even speed up through the workout, not slow down.

With an overview of each distance, Brian MacKenzie will now take you through the essential principles of the CFE plans.

Brian's Race-Specific Training Tips

5K

The 5K race isn't always given the respect it deserves in the larger running world. Do not make the mistake of underestimating this race. It demands maximum aerobic output from the opening gun right to the finish line. It is short on minutes but long on intensity.

Pacing is crucial—there just isn't time to make up for a poorly run first mile. Be sure to emphasize good form and a fast cadence. Setting and adhering to a good race pace plan for the 5K is critical. Let's say you are prepared to run 20 minutes flat for the 5K, but you want to break that. That means you are aiming to run at less than 6:24 per mile.

Your job, then, is to start fast but steady and aim to race your last mile faster than 6:24. If you get swept up in the frenzy of the start and run 6 minutes flat for the first mile, you'll be too cooked to even hold a 7-minute pace for the second mile. Rather, try to stick that first mile with a 6:24 split, hold the same pace through the second mile, then blast the final 1.125 miles with the best mile you have left in you. This is how you PR.

10K

The 10K is similar to the 5K in many ways, but it is a bit more forgiving of pacing errors because you have more time to recover from any early problems. As you go through the training plan, you'll train to avoid pacing errors, as the plan gives you a good understanding of what paces you can hold for different distances, such as 4 miles, 5 miles, and 6 miles.

In other words, the tempo and time trial runs should be used as stepping-stones to understanding paces you can hold at particular distances beyond the 5K. This will give you an excellent idea of the pace you should start out with in a 10K race. This training plan is designed to give you the strength to hold a fast speed through the end of the race, or what is called "even splits."

HALF-MARATHON

With the half-marathon, we start to get into the heart of one of the weaknesses I see in a lot of runners who come to our program: Their race pace for 5K and 10K races is not much different from their half-marathon pace.

That's a mistake. These are significantly different races and should be approached differently. The shorter races should be run faster, and the longer ones should be run slower to avoid bonking.

Still, you shouldn't ignore your 5K and 10K training. Why am I talking about your speed in race distances shorter than the race you want to train for? Because when you work in a way that improves your speed at race distances such as the 5K and 10K, you're going to be able to sustain a faster pace in long-distance races such as the half-marathon and up. As you train your anaerobic system and upgrade the speed at which you can run a 5K, you're going to drag your best half-marathon race pace along with it.

Here's how it works. Say you can run a 20-minute 5K race. It's safe to say that the pace you can hold in a 10K race is about 5 percent slower than that. Moving from the 10K to the half-marathon, one would begin to exhibit a larger deterioration in pace, but not by too much. A 10K at a pace of 6:40 per mile (95 percent of a 20-minute 5K pace) would yield a pace of right around 7:00 per mile, for a 1:32 half-marathon.

The first step to becoming a better racer is to recognize that you need a different plan for each race.

You can see that your pace in the shorter races is a predictor of the pace you can hold in longer races. The faster your short-race times, the faster your long-race times are likely to be.

If you are a little faster than this example, the difference between these numbers might be less, but not by much. If you are slower, these numbers will rise, and the difference between the race paces will increase. This explains why we focus on getting the shorter distances faster and faster as we "graduate" to the specified distance.

If you would like to run a 1:30 half, that requires you to run an average pace of about 7:00 per mile (1:30 half-marathon = 6:52 per mile average). Because you know that your pace will probably deteriorate as each mile clicks away, it is imperative that you learn where that deterioration starts to occur. This will be the key to your pacing plan for the half-marathon.

As your race distances increase, you need to take each time trial you've performed at different distances as a set of learning experiences. This will help you identify where to hold a pace and when to back off as the distances get longer.

Starting conservatively is never a mistake in a half-marathon, unless gold is on the line and it's worth the risk of blowing up. At that level you should understand exactly what pace you can and cannot get away with so that you can calculate the risk. But because 99.9 percent of us are not at that level, we need to start conservatively, hold steady, and finish fast. Ideally, we should be accelerating through the latter part of the race, achieving the much-sought-after "negative split."

MARATHON AND BEYOND

Long distances have become more and more popular in recent years. The marathon was once at the top of many runners' "bucket list," but now the ultramarathon—defined as anything longer than marathon distance but usually set at 50K, 50 miles, or 100 miles—has begun to take that place.

Much like the half-marathon, the pacing of these races depends largely on one's ability at the shorter distances. Most folks running marathons and ultramarathons don't tend to look to the shorter distances to help them build their ability to handle longer distances.

Instead, they continue to log slow miles and slowly push themselves toward their goals. Although there is nothing inherently wrong with that, it's an approach that's often less successful than CFE in delivering fast times with little postrun pain.

When approaching long distances, you can't really generate the same rate of energy output for a marathon as you can for a half-marathon. At mile 25 you will not feel the same as at mile 1. But it's not just a matter of energy output; by mile 25 you also will have broken down muscle and connective tissue.

There are two ways to buffer this deterioration: One is logging more slow miles, which requires more recovery time. Alternatively, you can speed up a bit with some of the shorter distances and implement a strength and conditioning program that has you recovering more quickly.

By now you know that the CFE approach is to do less volume at a higher intensity, with attention paid to strength, skill, and mobility improvement. An added benefit of CFE for ultrarunners, however, is that the lower weekly training volume in CFE programs also requires less time to execute. Instead of logging hours on the roads as you run one slow mile after the next, you will work breathlessly through your CFE workouts in a fraction of that time, with equal or better results.

One additional factor to be considered is the course. Most ultramarathons, and some marathons, are run on trails rather than roads, and some are notoriously difficult, with large climbs and descents. This kind of challenge requires a greater focus on strength and stabilization, and as a CFE athlete, you'll be especially well prepared to take on that challenge. Ultimately, that's the beauty of the CFE approach: The harder the challenge, the better prepared a CFE athlete will be to take it on.

5K TRAINING PLAN

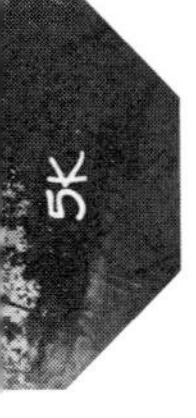

	LEVEL	M	T	W
WEEK 1	**BEGINNER**	CrossFit	**AM:** 45 min. drills 6–8 × 200 m/ rest 2:00 betw. each **PM:** CrossFit	CrossFit (run bias) or OFF
	INTERMEDIATE	CrossFit	**AM:** 30–45 min. drills 8–10 × 200 m/ rest 2:00 betw. each **PM:** CrossFit	CrossFit (run bias) or OFF
	ELITE	CrossFit	**AM:** 20–30 min. drills 10–12 × 200 m/ rest 1:30 betw. each **PM:** CrossFit	**PM:** 20–30 min drills 5K @ 85% of 10K race pace
WEEK 2	**BEGINNER**	CrossFit	AM: 30–45 min. drills 8–10 × 200 m/ rest 2:00 betw. each **PM:** CrossFit	CrossFit or OFF
	INTERMEDIATE	4 mile @ 80% of 5K TT pace	**AM:** CrossFit **PM:** 10–12 × 200 m/ rest 2:00 betw. each	CrossFit or OFF
	ELITE	CrossFit	**AM:** 20–30 min. drills 10–12 × 200 m/ easy 400 m betw. each **PM:** CrossFit	**AM:** 20–30 min drills 2 × 2 mi. as #1 @ 85–90% of best 2 mi. TT pace **PM:** CrossFit or OFF
WEEK 3	**BEGINNER**	CrossFit	**AM:** 30–45 min. drills 8–10 × 200 m/ rest 1:30 betw. each **PM:** CrossFit	CrossFit (run bias) or OFF
	INTERMEDIATE	CrossFit/CFE S & C Recovery*/OFF	**AM:** 20–30 min. drills 10–12 × 200 m/ rest 1:30 betw. each **PM:** CrossFit	CrossFit (run bias) or OFF
	ELITE	CrossFit/CFE S & C Recovery/OFF	**AM:** 20–30 min. drills 5–6 × 400 m/ rest 2:00 betw. each **PM:** CrossFit	CrossFit

T	F	S	S
45 min. drills 2–3 × 800 m/ rest 3:00 betw. each	CrossFit or OFF	CrossFit or OFF	30 min. drills 2 mi. TT
30–45 min. drills 4–5 × 800 m/ rest 2:30 betw. each	CrossFit or OFF	30 min. drills 2 × 1 mi. TT/ rest 5 min. betw.	CrossFit
20–30 min. drills 6–8 × 800 m/ rest 2:30 betw. each	CrossFit or OFF	**AM:** CrossFit or OFF **PM:** 15–20 min drills 5K @ 80% of 5K race pace	15 min. drills 2 × 2 mi. TT/ rest 5:00–7:00 betw. each
45 min. drills 3–4 × 800 m/ rest 3:00 betw. each	CrossFit (run bias) or OFF	30 min. drills 3 × 1 mi. @ 90% of 2 mi. TT pace/ rest 5 min. betw. each	CrossFit or OFF
30–45 min. drills 4–5 × 800 m/ rest 2:15 betw. each	CrossFit or OFF	CrossFit	15–20 min. drills 5K @ 80% of added 1 mi. TT pace (2 mi. time @ 80%)
20–30 min. drills 6–8 × 800 m/ rest 2:15 betw. each	CrossFit or OFF	**AM:** 30 min. drills Tabata sprints **PM:** CrossFit or OFF	15 min. drills 5K @ 80% of 5K race pace
30–45 min. drills 3–4 × 800 m/ rest 2:45 betw. each	CrossFit or OFF	CrossFit or OFF	30 min. drills 2 mi. TT
30–45 min. drills 6–8 × 800 m/ easy 600 m betw. each	CrossFit or OFF	15–20 min. drills 2 mi. TT	CrossFit or OFF
30–45 min. drills 6–8 × 800 m/ easy 400 m betw. each	CrossFit (run bias) or OFF	15–20 min. drills 2 mi. TT	**AM:** 30 min. drills 3 × 1 mi. @ 5K race pace/rest 3:00 betw. each **PM:** CrossFit or OFF

CONTINUED

5K TRAINING PLAN *continued*

WEEK	LEVEL	M	T	W
WEEK 4	**BEGINNER**	CrossFit/CFE S & C Recovery/OFF	**AM:** 30–45 min. drills 10–12 × 200 m/ rest 1:30 betw. each **PM:** CrossFit	CrossFit (run bias)
	INTERMEDIATE	CrossFit	**AM:** 20–30 min. drills 4–6 × 400 m/ easy 200 m betw. each **PM:** CrossFit	CrossFit
	ELITE	CrossFit/CFE S & C Recovery/OFF	**AM:** 20–30 min. drills 6–8 × 400 m/ easy 200 m betw. each **PM:** CrossFit	CrossFit
WEEK 5	**BEGINNER**	CrossFit	**AM:** 30–45 min. drills 4–6 × 400 m/ rest 2:00 betw. each **PM:** CrossFit	CrossFit
	INTERMEDIATE	CrossFit/CFE S & C Recovery/OFF	**AM:** 20–30 min. drills 4–6 × 400 m/ rest 1:45 betw. each **PM:** CrossFit	CrossFit (run bias)
	ELITE	CrossFit/CFE S & C Recovery/OFF	**AM:** 20–30 min. drills 6–8 × 400 m/ rest 1:30 betw. each **PM:** CrossFit	CrossFit (run bias)
WEEK 6	**BEGINNER**	CrossFit	**AM:** 30–45 min. drills 4–6 × 400 m/ rest 1:45 betw. each **PM:** CrossFit	CrossFit
	INTERMEDIATE	CrossFit/CFE S & C Recovery/OFF	**AM:** 20–30 min. drills 6–8 × 400 m/ easy 200 m betw. each PM: CrossFit	CrossFit
	ELITE	CrossFit/CFE S & C Recovery/OFF	**AM:** 20–30 min. drills 8–10 × 400 m/ easy 200 m betw. each **PM:** CrossFit	CrossFit (run bias)

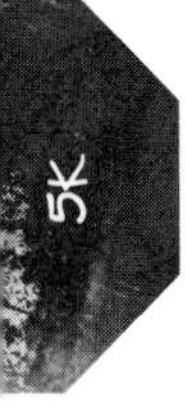

T	F	S	S
30–45 min. drills 4–5 × 800 m/ rest 2:45 betw. each	CrossFit or OFF	30 min. drills 2 × 2 mi. @ 85% of 2 mi. TT pace	CrossFit or OFF
30–45 min. drills 3–4 × 1000 m/ rest 3:00 betw. each	CrossFit (run bias) or OFF	**AM:** 30 min. drills Tabata sprints **PM:** CrossFit or OFF	15–20 min. drills 1 mi. TT/rest 5–8 min. + 2 × 2 mi. @ 90% of 2 mi. TT pace
30–45 min. drills 4–6 × 1000 m/ rest 2:30 betw. each	15–20 min. drills 5K @ 80% of 2 mi. TT pace	CrossFit or OFF	30 min. drills 3 × 2 mi. @ 5K race pace/rest 3:00–5:00 betw. each
30–45 min. drills 4–5 × 800 m/ rest 2:30 betw. each	CrossFit or OFF	CrossFit	20–30 min. drills 3 × 1 mi. TT/rest 5:00–8:00 betw. each
30–45 min. drills 4–5 × 1000 m/ easy 600 m betw. each	CrossFit	CrossFit or OFF	15–20 min. drills 5K @ 80% of 2 mi. TT pace
30–45 min. drills 5–6 × 1000 m/ easy 600 m betw. each	CrossFit	15–20 min. drills 5K @ 80% of 2 mi. TT pace	30 min. drills 4 × 1 mi. @ 90%+ of 2 mi. TT pace/rest 3:00–5:00 betw. each
30–45 min. drills 5–6 × 800 m/ rest 2:30 betw. each	CrossFit or OFF	30 min. drills 2 × 2 mi. TT/rest 10:00 betw. each	CrossFit/CFE S & C Recovery/OFF
30–45 min. drills 4–5 × 1000 m/ rest 3:00 betw. each	CrossFit (run bias) or OFF	20–30 min. drills 5K @ 85% of 5K race pace	**AM:** 30 min. drills Tabata sprints **PM:** CrossFit or OFF
30–45 min. drills 5–6 × 1000 m/ rest 2:15 betw. each	CrossFit	15–20 min. drills 5K @ 90% of 5K race pace	30 min. drills 3 × 1 mi. @ 90%+ of 2 mi. TT pace/rest 3:00–5:00 betw. each

CONTINUED

5K TRAINING PLAN *continued*

	LEVEL	M	T	W
WEEK 7	BEGINNER	CrossFit	**AM:** 30–45 min. drills 4–6 × 400 m/ rest 1:30 betw. each **PM:** CrossFit	CrossFit
	INTERMEDIATE	CrossFit/CFE S & C Recovery/OFF	**AM:** 20–30 min. drills 6–8 × 400 m/ rest 1:15 betw. each **PM:** CrossFit	CrossFit (run bias)
	ELITE	CrossFit/CFE S & C Recovery/OFF	**AM:** 20–30 min. drills 8–10 × 400 m/ rest 1:15 betw. each **PM:** CrossFit	CrossFit (run bias)
WEEK 8	BEGINNER	CrossFit	**AM:** 30–45 min. drills 8 × 200 m/ easy 200 m betw. each **PM:** CrossFit	CrossFit (run bias)
	INTERMEDIATE	CrossFit/CFE S & C Recovery/OFF	**AM:** 20–30 min. drills 10 × 200 m/ easy 200 m betw. each **PM:** CrossFit	CrossFit (run bias)
	ELITE	CrossFit/CFE S & C Recovery/OFF	**AM:** 20–30 min. drills 10 × 200 m/ easy 200 m betw. each **PM:** CrossFit	CrossFit (run bias)
TAPER WEEK	ALL LEVELS	**AM:** Squat 5 × 3 or 5 × 5 at 80–90% of usual weight **PM:** 8–12 × 200 m/ rest 2:00 betw. each. Hold paces you held at start of program. Focus on technique.	Easy 30 min. run	Easy walking or OFF

200s: 98+ cadence   400s: 98+ cadence   800s: 96+ cadence   1000s: 95+ cadence
1200s: 95+ cadence   1 mi.: 95+ cadence   2 mi.: 95+ cadence   5K: 95+ cadence
You should be able to maintain the same relative pace for each of these intervals.

T	F	S	S
30–45 min. drills 3–4 × 1000 m/ easy 600 m betw. each	CrossFit (run bias)	OFF	30 min. drills 2 × 2 mi. TT/rest 5:00–7:00 betw.
30–45 min. drills 5–6 × 1000 m/ easy 600 m betw. each	CrossFit	20–30 min. drills 5K @ 85% of 5K race pace	**AM:** 30 min. drills Tabata sprints **PM:** CrossFit or OFF
30–45 min. drills 6–7 × 1000 m/ easy 400 m betw. each	**AM:** CrossFit **PM:** 15 min. drills Tabata sprints	15–20 min. drills 5K @ 90% of 5K race pace	**AM:** 30 min. drills Tabata sprints **PM:** CrossFit or OFF
30–45 min. drills 5 × 800 m/ rest 3:30 betw. each	CrossFit	OFF	30 min. drills 3 × 1.5 mi. TT/rest 5:00–7:00 betw. each
30–45 min. drills 4 × 1000 m/ rest 3:00 betw. each	**AM:** 30 min. drills Tabata sprints **PM:** CrossFit or OFF	CrossFit or OFF	15–20 min. drills 2 × 2 mi. TT/rest 5:00–7:00 betw.
30–45 min. drills 5 × 1000 m/ rest 2:15 betw. each	**AM:** CrossFit **PM:** 15 min. drills Tabata sprints	15–20 min. drills 3 × 2 mi. TT/rest 5:00–7:00 betw. each	**AM:** 30 min. drills Tabata sprints **PM:** CrossFit or OFF
AM: 3–5 RFT of 5 pull-ups, 10 push-ups, 15 squats **PM:** 3–4 × 400 m @ 70% effort, walk 200 m betw. each. Focus on technique.	Easy walking or OFF	RACE or easy 20–30 min. run	RACE + CFE S & C Recovery

**The CFE S & C recovery circuit may be found in Chapter 5, page 127.*

10K TRAINING PLAN

	LEVEL	M	T	W
WEEK 1	BEGINNER	CrossFit	**AM:** 45 min. drills 6–8 × 200 m/ rest 2:00 betw. each **PM:** CrossFit	CrossFit (run bias) or OFF
	INTERMEDIATE	CrossFit	**AM:** 30–45 min. drills 8–10 × 200 m/ rest 2:00 betw. each **PM:** CrossFit	CrossFit (run bias) or OFF
	ELITE	CrossFit	**AM:** 20–30 min. drills 10–12 × 200 m/ easy 400 m betw. each **PM:** CrossFit	**PM:** 20–30 min. drills 5K @ 85% of 10K race pace
WEEK 2	BEGINNER	CrossFit	**AM:** 30–45 min. drills 8–10 × 200 m/ rest 2:00 betw. each **PM:** CrossFit	CrossFit or OFF
	INTERMEDIATE	4 mile @ 80% of 5K TT pace	**AM:** CrossFit **PM:** 5–6 × 300 m/ rest 2:00 betw. each	CrossFit or OFF
	ELITE	CrossFit	AM: 20–30 min. drills 6–8 × 300 m/ rest 1:30 betw. each **PM:** CrossFit	**AM:** 20–30 min. drills 5K @ 80% of 5K race pace **PM:** CrossFit or OFF
WEEK 3	BEGINNER	CrossFit	**AM:** 30–45 min. drills 5–6 × 300 m/ rest 2:00 betw. each **PM:** CrossFit	CrossFit (run bias) or OFF
	INTERMEDIATE	CrossFit/CFE S & C Recovery*/OFF	**AM:** 20–30 min. drills 5–6 × 300 m/ easy 400 m betw. each **PM:** CrossFit	CrossFit (run bias) or OFF
	ELITE	CrossFit/CFE S & C Recovery/OFF	**AM:** 20–30 min. drils 5K @ 85% 5K race pace w/3 × 400 m @ race pace in middle **PM:** CrossFit	CrossFit

T	F	S	S
45 min. drills 2–3 × 800 m/ rest 3:00 betw. each	CrossFit or OFF	CrossFit or OFF	30 min. drills 2 mi. TT
30–45 min. drills 4–5 × 800 m/ rest 2:30 betw. each	CrossFit or OFF	30 min. drills 5K TT	CrossFit
20–30 min. drills 6–8 × 800 m/ rest 2:30 betw. each	CrossFit or OFF	**AM:** CrossFit or OFF **PM:** 15–20 min. drills 5K @ 80% of 5K race pace	15 min. drills 5K TT, same course as yesterday
45 min. drills 3–4 × 800 m/ rest 3:00 betw. each	CrossFit (run bias) or OFF	30 min. drills 5K @ 80% of 2 mi. TT pace	CrossFit or OFF
30–45 min. drills 4–5 × 800 m/ easy 600 m betw. each	CrossFit or OFF	CrossFit	15–20 min. drills 5K @ 80% of 5K TT pace
20–30 min. drills 6–8 × 800 m/ easy 600 m betw. each	CrossFit or OFF	**AM:** 30 min. drills Tabata sprints **PM:** CrossFit or OFF	15 min. drills 5 mi. @ 85% of 10K race pace
30–45 min. drills 3–4 × 800 m/ rest 2:45 betw. each	CrossFit or OFF	CrossFit or OFF	30 min. drills 4 mi. TT
30–45 min. drills 6–8 × 800 m/ rest 2:30 betw. each	CrossFit or OFF	15–20 min. drills 4 mi. TT	CrossFit or OFF
30–45 min. drills 6–8 × 800 m/ rest 2:00 betw. each	CrossFit (run bias) or OFF	15–20 min. drills 4 mi. TT	**AM:** 30 min. drills 5K @ 80% of 10K race pace **PM:** CrossFit or OFF

CONTINUED

10K TRAINING PLAN *continued*

	LEVEL	M	T	W
WEEK 4	**BEGINNER**	CrossFit/CFE S & C Recovery/OFF	**AM:** 30–45 min. drills 6 × 300 m/ rest 1:45 betw. each **PM:** CrossFit	CrossFit (run bias)
	INTERMEDIATE	CrossFit	**AM:** 20–30 min. drills 4–6 × 400 m/ rest 2:00 betw. each **PM:** CrossFit	CrossFit
	ELITE	CrossFit/CFE S & C Recovery/OFF	**AM:** 20–30 min. drills 6–8 × 400 m/ easy 400 m betw. each **PM:** CrossFit	CrossFit
WEEK 5	**BEGINNER**	CrossFit	**AM:** 30–45 min. drills 4–5 × 400 m/ rest 2:00 betw. each **PM:** CrossFit	CrossFit
	INTERMEDIATE	CrossFit/CFE S & C Recovery/OFF	**AM:** 20–30 min. drills 4–6 × 400 m/ easy 300 m betw. each **PM:** CrossFit	CrossFit (run bias)
	ELITE	CrossFit/CFE S & C Recovery/OFF	**AM:** 20–30 min. drills 5 mi. @ 85% of 4 mi. TT pace **PM:** CrossFit	CrossFit (run bias)
WEEK 6	**BEGINNER**	CrossFit	**AM:** 30–45 min. drills 4–6 × 400 m/ easy 400 m betw. each **PM:** CrossFit	CrossFit
	INTERMEDIATE	CrossFit/CFE S & C Recovery/OFF	**AM:** 20–30 min. drills 6–8 × 400 m/ easy 300 m betw. each **PM:** CrossFit	CrossFit
	ELITE	CrossFit/CFE S & C Recovery/OFF	**AM:** 20–30 min. drills 8–10 × 400 m/ easy 300 m betw. each **PM:** CrossFit	CrossFit (run bias)

T	F	S	S
30–45 min. drills 4–5 × 800 m/ rest 2:45 betw. each	CrossFit or OFF	30 min. drills 2 × 2 mi. @ 90% of 4 mi. TT pace	CrossFit or OFF
30–45 min. drills 3–4 × 1000 m/ easy 600 m betw. each	CrossFit (run bias) or OFF	**AM:** 30 min. drills Tabata sprints **PM:** CrossFit or OFF	15–20 min. drills 1 mi. TT/rest 5–8 min. 2 × 2 mi. @ 85%+ of 1 mi. TT pace
30 min. drills 4–5 mi. @ 85% of 4 mi. TT pace	CrossFit or OFF	CrossFit or OFF	30 min. drills 3 × 2 mi. @ 5K race pace/rest 3:00–5:00 betw. each
30–45 min. drills 4–5 × 800 m/ rest 2:30 betw. each	CrossFit or OFF	CrossFit	20–30 min. drills 5 mi. TT
30–45 min. drills 4–5 × 1000 m/ rest 3:00 betw. each	CrossFit	CrossFit or OFF	15–20 min. drills 5 mi. TT
30–45 min. drills 5–6 × 1000 m/ easy 400 m betw. each	CrossFit	15–20 min. drills 5K @ 80% of 2 mi. TT pace	30 min. drills 4 × 1 mi. @ 90%+ of 2 mi. TT pace/rest 3:00–5:00 betw. each
30–45 min. drills 5–6 × 800 m/ rest 2:30 betw. each	CrossFit or OFF	30 min. drills 2 × 2 mi. TT/ rest 10:00 betw. each	CrossFit/CFE S & C Recovery/OFF
30–45 min. drills 4–5 × 1000 m/ rest 3:00 betw. each	CrossFit (run bias) or OFF	20–30 min. drills 5K @ 85% of 5K race pace	**AM:** 30 min. drills Tabata sprints **PM:** CrossFit or OFF
30–45 min. drills 5–6 × 1000 m/ rest 2:15 betw. each	CrossFit	15–20 min. drills 10K @ 90% of 5K race pace	**AM:** 30 min. drills Tabata sprints **PM:** CrossFit or OFF

CONTINUED

10K TRAINING PLAN *continued*

	LEVEL	M	T	W
WEEK 7	BEGINNER	CrossFit	**AM:** 30–45 min. drills 4–6 × 400 m/ easy 400 m betw. each **PM:** CrossFit	CrossFit
	INTERMEDIATE	CrossFit/CFE S & C Recovery/OFF	**AM:** 20–30 min. drills 6–8 × 400 m/ rest 1:15 betw. each **PM:** CrossFit	CrossFit (run bias)
	ELITE	CrossFit/CFE S & C Recovery/OFF	**AM:** 30 min. drills 6–7 × 1000 m/ rest 2:15 betw. each **PM:** CrossFit	CrossFit (run bias)
WEEK 8	BEGINNER	CrossFit	**AM:** 30–45 min. drills 4 × 400 m/ easy 400 m betw. each **PM:** CrossFit	CrossFit (run bias)
	INTERMEDIATE	CrossFit/CFE S & C Recovery/OFF	**AM:** 20–30 min. drills 6 × 300 m/ easy 300 m betw. each **PM:** CrossFit	CrossFit (run bias)
	ELITE	CrossFit/CFE S & C Recovery/OFF	**AM:** 20–30 min. drills 6 × 400 m/ easy 200 m betw. each **PM:** CrossFit	CrossFit (run bias)
TAPER WEEK	ALL LEVELS	**AM:** Squat 5 × 3 or 5 × 5 at 80–90% of usual weight **PM:** 8–12 × 200 m/ rest 2:00 betw. each. Hold paces you held at start of program. Focus on technique.	Easy 30 min. run	Easy walking or OFF

200s: *98+ cadence* *400s:* *98+ cadence* *800s:* *96+ cadence* *1000s:* *95+ cadence*
1200s: *95+ cadence* *1 mi.:* *95+ cadence* *2 mi.:* *95+ cadence* *5K:* *95+ cadence*
You should be able to maintain the same relative pace for each of these intervals.

10K

T	F	S	S
30–45 min. drills 3–4 × 1000 m/ rest 3:30 betw. each	CrossFit (run bias)	OFF	30 min. drills 5 mi. TT
30–45 min. drills 5–6 × 1000 m/ easy 400 betw. each	CrossFit	20–30 min. drills 10K @ 80% of 5K race pace	**AM:** 30 min. drills Tabata sprints **PM:** CrossFit or OFF
30 min. drills 4 mi. @ 85% of 4 mi. TT pace	**AM:** CrossFit **PM:** 15 min. drills Tabata sprints	15–20 min. drills 2 × 3 mi. @ 90%+ of 5K race pace/ rest 5:00–10:00 betw. each	**AM:** 30 min. drills Tabata sprints **PM:** CrossFit or OFF
30–45 min. drills 5 × 800 m/ rest 3:30 betw. each	CrossFit	OFF	30 min. drills 5K @ 90%+ of 5K race pace
30–45 min. drills 4 × 1000 m/ rest 3:00 betw. each	**AM:** 30 min. drills Tabata sprints **PM:** CrossFit or OFF	CrossFit or OFF	15–20 min. drills 5 mi. @ 90%+ of 4 mi. TT pace
30–45 min. drills 5 × 1000 m/ rest 3:00 betw. each	**AM:** CrossFit **PM:** 15 min. drills Tabata sprints	15–20 min. drills 2 × 3 mi. TT/rest 5:00–10:00 betw.	**AM:** 30 min. drills Tabata sprints **PM:** CrossFit or OFF
AM: 3–5 RFT of 5 pull-ups, 10 push-ups, 15 squats **PM:** 3–4 × 400 m @ 70% effort, walk 200 m betw. each. Focus on technique.	Easy walking or OFF	RACE or easy 20–30 min. run	RACE + CFE S & C Recovery

**The CFE S & C recovery circuit may be found in Chapter 5, page 127.*

HALF-MARATHON TRAINING PLAN

	LEVEL	M	T	W
WEEK 1	BEGINNER	CrossFit	**AM:** 45 min. drills 6–8 × 200 m/ rest 2:00 betw. each **PM:** CrossFit	CrossFit (run bias) or OFF
	INTERMEDIATE	CrossFit	**AM:** 30–45 min. drills 8–10 × 200 m/ rest 2:00 betw. each **PM:** CrossFit	CrossFit (run bias) or OFF
	ELITE	CrossFit	**AM:** 20–30 min. drills 10–12 × 200 m/ rest 1:30 betw. each **PM:** CrossFit	**PM:** 20–30 min. drills 5K @ 85% of 10K race pace
WEEK 2	BEGINNER	CrossFit	**AM:** 30–45 min. drills 8–10 × 200 m/ rest 1:30 betw. each **PM:** CrossFit	CrossFit or OFF
	INTERMEDIATE	5K @ 80% of 5K TT pace	**AM:** CrossFit **PM:** 4–5 × 400 m/ rest 2:00 betw. each	CrossFit or OFF
	ELITE	CrossFit	**AM:** 20–30 min. drills 5–6 × 400 m/ easy 400 m betw. each **PM:** CrossFit	**AM:** 20–30 min. drills 5 mi. @ 80% of 5K race pace **PM:** CrossFit or OFF
WEEK 3	BEGINNER	CrossFit	**AM:** 30–45 min. drills 4–5 × 400 m/ rest 2:00 betw. each **PM:** CrossFit	CrossFit (run bias) or OFF
	INTERMEDIATE	CrossFit/CFE S & C Recovery*/OFF	**AM:** 20–30 min. drills 4–5 × 400 m/ rest 1:30 betw. each **PM:** CrossFit	CrossFit (run bias) or OFF
	ELITE	CrossFit/CFE S & C Recovery/OFF	**AM:** 20–30 min. drills 5K @ 85% 5K race pace w/ 3 × 400 m @ race pace in middle of 5K **PM:** CrossFit	CrossFit

T	F	S	S
45 min. drills 2–3 × 800 m/ rest 3:00 betw. each	CrossFit or OFF	CrossFit or OFF	30 min. drills 5K TT
30–45 min. drills 4–5 × 800 m/ rest 2:30 betw. each	CrossFit or OFF	30 min. drills 5K TT	CrossFit
20–30 min. drills 6–8 × 800 m/ rest 2:30 betw. each	CrossFit or OFF	**AM:** CrossFit or OFF **PM:** 15–20 min. drills 5K @ 80% of 5K race pace	15 min. drills 5K TT, same course as yesterday
45 min. drills 3 × 800 m/ rest 3:00 betw. each	CrossFit (run bias) or OFF	30 min. drills 4 mi. @ 80% of 10K race pace	CrossFit or OFF
30–45 min. drills 4–5 × 800 m/ rest 2:30 betw. each	CrossFit or OFF	15–20 min. drills 5K @ 80% of 5K TT pace	CrossFit (run bias)
20–30 min. drills 6–8 × 800 m/ rest 2:30 betw. each	CrossFit or OFF	**AM:** 45 min. drills **PM:** CrossFit or OFF	15 min. drills 5 mi. @ 90% of 10K race pace
30–45 min. drills 3–4 × 800 m/ rest 2:45 betw. each	CrossFit or OFF	CrossFit or OFF	30 min. drills 4 mi. TT
30–45 min. drills 6–8 × 800 m/ easy 400 m betw. each	CrossFit or OFF	15–20 min. drills 4 mi. TT	CrossFit (run bias) @ 80–90% effort or OFF
30–45 min. drills 6–8 × 800 m/ easy 400 m betw. each	CrossFit (run bias) or OFF	15–20 min. drills 10K TT	**AM:** 30 min. drills 5K @ 80% of 10K race pace **PM:** CrossFit or OFF

CONTINUED

HALF-MARATHON TRAINING PLAN *continued*

	LEVEL	M	T	W
WEEK 4	BEGINNER	CrossFit/CFE S & C Recovery/OFF	**AM:** 30–45 min. drills 8 × 300 m/ easy 300 m betw. each **PM:** CrossFit	CrossFit (run bias)
	INTERMEDIATE	CrossFit	**AM:** 20–30 min. drills 5–6 × 400 m/ easy 300 m betw. each **PM:** CrossFit	CrossFit
	ELITE	CrossFit/CFE S & C Recovery/OFF	**AM:** 20–30 min. drills 6–8 × 400 m/ easy 400 m betw. each **PM:** CrossFit	CrossFit
WEEK 5	BEGINNER	OFF	**AM:** 30–45 min. drills 5–6 × 400 m/ easy 300 m betw. each **PM:** CrossFit	CrossFit
	INTERMEDIATE	CrossFit/CFE S & C Recovery/OFF	**AM:** 20–30 min. drills 4–6 × 400 m/ rest 1:45 betw. each **PM:** CrossFit	CrossFit (run bias)
	ELITE	CrossFit/CFE S & C Recovery/OFF	**AM:** 20–30 min. drills 5 mi. @ 85% of 4 mi. TT pace/ rest 1:30 betw. each **PM:** CrossFit	CrossFit (run bias)
WEEK 6	BEGINNER	CrossFit	**AM:** 30–45 min. drills 5–6 × 400 m/ easy 300 m betw. each **PM:** CrossFit	CrossFit
	INTERMEDIATE	CrossFit/CFE S & C Recovery/OFF	**AM:** 20–30 min. drills 5K @ 90% of 5K race pace **PM:** CrossFit	CrossFit
	ELITE	CrossFit/CFE S & C Recovery/OFF	**AM:** 20–30 min. drills 8–10 × 400 m/ easy 300 m betw. each **PM:** CrossFit	CrossFit (run bias)

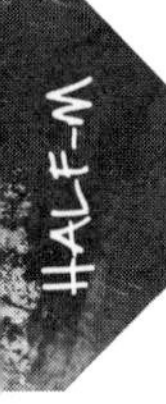

T	F	S	S
30–45 min. drills 4–5 × 800 m/ rest 2:45 betw. each	CrossFit or OFF	**AM:** 30 min. drills 5K @ 80% of 5K race pace **PM:** 15 min. drills 5K @ 85%+ of 5K race pace	CrossFit @ 80% effort or OFF
30–45 min. drills 3–4 × 1000 m/ rest 3:00 betw. each	CrossFit (run bias) or OFF	**AM:** 30 min. drills Tabata sprints **PM:** CrossFit or OFF	15–20 min. drills 10K TT
30 min. drills 4–5 mi. @ 85% of 5K race pace	CrossFit or OFF	CrossFit or OFF	30 min. drills 3 × 5K @ 80%+ of 5K race pace, split morning, noon, evening
30–45 min. drills 4–5 × 800 m/ rest 2:30 betw. each	CrossFit or OFF	CrossFit	20–30 min. drills 10K TT
30–45 min. drills 4–5 × 1000 m/ easy 600 m betw. each	CrossFit	CrossFit or OFF	15–20 min. drills 5 mi. @ 85% of 10K TT pace
30–45 min. drills 5–6 × 1000 m/ easy 600 m betw. each	CrossFit	15–20 min. drills 3–4 × 1 mi. @ 5K race pace/ rest 3:00 betw. each	30 min. drills 8 mi. @ 85% of 10K race pace
30–45 min. drills 5–6 × 800 m/ rest 2:30 betw. each	CrossFit or OFF	30 min. drills 2 × 5K TT/ rest 10:00 betw.	CrossFit/CFE S & C Recovery/OFF
30–45 min. drills 4–5 × 1000 m/ rest 3:00 betw. each	CrossFit (run bias) or OFF	20–30 min. drills 5K @ 85% of 5K race pace	**AM:** 30 min. drills Tabata sprints **PM:** CrossFit or OFF
30–45 min. drills 5–6 × 1000 m/ rest 2:30 betw. each	CrossFit	15–20 min. drills 15K @ 80% of 10K race pace	**AM:** 30 min. drills Tabata sprints **PM:** CrossFit or OFF

HALF-M

CONTINUED

HALF-MARATHON TRAINING PLAN *continued*

	LEVEL	M	T	W
WEEK 7	BEGINNER	CrossFit	**AM:** 30–45 min. drills 4 × 600 m/ easy 400 m betw. each **PM:** CrossFit	CrossFit
	INTERMEDIATE	CrossFit/CFE S & C Recovery/OFF	**AM:** 20–30 min. drills 6–8 × 600 m/ rest 1:30 betw. each **PM:** CrossFit	CrossFit (run bias)
	ELITE	CrossFit/CFE S & C Recovery/OFF	**AM:** 30 min. drills 6–7 × 1000 m/ rest 2:30 betw. each **PM:** CrossFit	CrossFit (run bias)
WEEK 8	BEGINNER	CrossFit	**AM:** 30–45 min. drills 5–6 × 600 m/ easy 400 m betw. each **PM:** CrossFit	CrossFit (run bias)
	INTERMEDIATE	CrossFit/CFE S & C Recovery/OFF	**AM:** 20–30 min. drills 6–8 × 600 m/ easy 400 m betw. each **PM:** CrossFit	CrossFit (run bias)
	ELITE	CrossFit/CFE S & C Recovery/OFF	**AM:** 20 min. drills 10K @ 80% of 10K race pace **PM:** CrossFit	CrossFit (run bias)
WEEK 9	BEGINNER	CrossFit	**AM:** 30–45 min. drills 5–6 × 400 m/ rest 1:30 betw. each **PM:** CrossFit	CrossFit (run bias)
	INTERMEDIATE	CrossFit/CFE S & C Recovery/OFF	**AM:** 20–30 min. drills 6–8 × 400 m/ rest 1:30 betw. each **PM:** CrossFit	CrossFit (run bias)
	ELITE	CrossFit/CFE S & C Recovery/ OFF	**AM:** 20 min. drills 8–10 × 400 m/ easy 300 m betw. each **PM:** CrossFit	CrossFit (run bias)

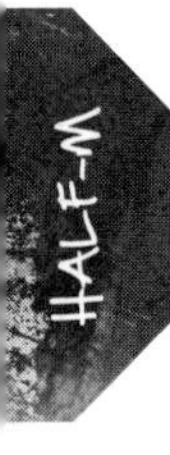

T	F	S	S
30–45 min. drills 3–4 × 1000 m/ rest 3:30 betw. each	CrossFit (run bias)	OFF	30 min. drills 10K @ 80% of 10K race pace
30–45 min. drills 5–6 × 1000 m/ easy 600 m betw. each	CrossFit	20–30 min. drills 10K @ 80% of 5K race pace	**AM:** 30 min. drills Tabata sprints **PM:** CrossFit or OFF
30 min. drills 5 mi. @ 85% of 10K race pace	**AM:** CrossFit **PM:** 15 min. drills Tabata sprints	15–20 min. drills 3 × 3 mi. @ 90%+ of 5K race pace/rest 5:00–10:00 betw. each	**AM:** 30 min. drills Tabata sprints **PM:** CrossFit or OFF
30–45 min. drills 3–4 × 1000 m/ rest 3:00 betw. each	CrossFit	OFF	30 min. drills 15K TT
30–45 min. drills 5–6 × 1000 m/ rest 3:00 betw. each	**AM:** 30 min. drills Tabata sprints **PM:** CrossFit or OFF	CrossFit or OFF	15–20 min. drills 10 mi. TT
30–45 min. drills 5–6 × 1000 m/ rest 2:30 betw. each	**AM:** CrossFit **PM:** 15 min. drills Tabata sprints	15–20 min. drills 10 mi. TT	30 min. drills 4 × 1 mi. @ 80% of 5K race pace/ rest 3:00 betw. each
30–45 min. drills 3–4 × 1000 m/ easy 600 m betw. each	CrossFit	OFF	30 min. drills 8 mi. @ 85% of 15K TT pace
30–45 min. drills 5–6 × 1000 m/ easy 600 m betw. each	**AM:** 30 min. drills Tabata sprints **PM:** CrossFit or OFF	CrossFit or OFF	15–20 min. drills 10 mi. @ 80% of 10 mi. TT pace
30–45 min. drills 5–6 × 1000 m/ rest 2:30 betw. each	**AM:** CrossFit **PM:** 15 min. drills Tabata sprints	15–20 min. drills 12 mi. @ 80% of 10 mi. TT	30 min. drills 5K @ 90%+ of 5K race pace

CONTINUED

HALF-MARATHON TRAINING PLAN *continued*

	LEVEL	M	T	W
WEEK 10	BEGINNER	CrossFit	**AM:** 30–45 min. drills 5–6 × 600 m/ easy 300 m betw. each **PM:** CrossFit	CrossFit (run bias)
	INTERMEDIATE	CrossFit/CFE S & C Recovery/OFF	**AM:** 20–30 min. drills 6–8 × 600 m/ easy 300 m betw. each **PM:** CrossFit	CrossFit (run bias)
	ELITE	CrossFit/CFE S & C Recovery/OFF	**AM:** 20 min. drills 10K @ 80% of 10K race pace **PM:** CrossFit or OFF	CrossFit (run bias)
TAPER WEEK	ALL LEVELS	**AM:** Squat 5 × 3 or 5 × 5 at 80–90% of usual weight **PM:** 8–12 × 200 m/ rest 2:00 betw. each. Hold paces you held at start of program. Focus on technique.	Easy 30 min. run	Easy walking or OFF

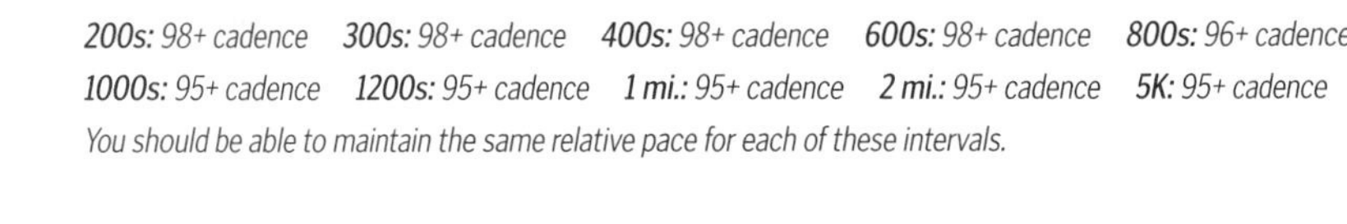

200s: *98+ cadence* *300s:* *98+ cadence* *400s:* *98+ cadence* *600s:* *98+ cadence* *800s:* *96+ cadence*
1000s: *95+ cadence* *1200s:* *95+ cadence* *1 mi.:* *95+ cadence* *2 mi.:* *95+ cadence* *5K:* *95+ cadence*
You should be able to maintain the same relative pace for each of these intervals.

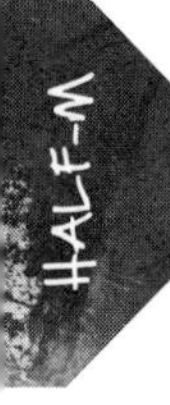

T	F	S	S
30–45 min. drills 2 × 200 m/rest 1:30 + 2 × 400 m/rest 1:30 + 2 × 1000 m/rest 3:00 betw. each	CrossFit	OFF	30 min. drills 8 mi. @ 85% of 15K TT pace
30–45 min. drills 2 × 200 m/rest 1:30 + 2 × 400 m/rest 1:30 + 3 × 1000 m/rest 3:00 betw. each	CrossFit (run bias) or OFF	15–20 min. drills 10K @ 80% of 10K race pace	15–20 min. drills 3 × 5K @ 80–90% of 5K race pace/ rest 10:00–15:00 betw. each
30–45 min. drills 3 × 200 m/rest 1:30 + 3 × 400 m/rest 1:30 + 4 × 1000 m/rest 3:00 betw. each	CrossFit (run bias) or OFF	15–20 min. drills 10 mi. @ 80% of 10 mi. TT pace	30 min. drills 10K @ 90%+ of 10K race pace
AM: 3–5 RFT of 5 pull-ups, 10 push-ups, 15 squats **PM:** 3–4 × 400 m @ 70% effort, walk 200 m betw. each. Focus on technique.	Easy walking or OFF	RACE or easy 20–30 min. run	RACE + CFE S & C Recovery

The CFE S & C recovery circuit may be found in Chapter 5, page 127.

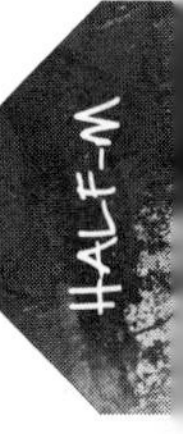

MARATHON TRAINING PLAN

	LEVEL	M	T	W
WEEK 1	BEGINNER	CrossFit	**AM:** 45 min. drills 6–8 × 200 m/ rest 2:00 betw. each **PM:** CrossFit	CrossFit (run bias) or OFF
	INTERMEDIATE	CrossFit	**AM:** 30–45 min. drills 8–10 × 200 m/ rest 2:00 betw. each **PM:** CrossFit	CrossFit (run bias) or OFF
	ELITE	CrossFit	**AM:** 20–30 min. drills 10–12 × 200 m/ easy 300 m betw. each **PM:** CrossFit	20–30 min. drills 5K @ 85% of 10K race pace
WEEK 2	BEGINNER	CrossFit	**AM:** 30–45 min. drills 8–10 × 200 m/ rest 1:30 betw. each **PM:** CrossFit	CrossFit or OFF
	INTERMEDIATE	5K @ 80% of 5K TT pace	**AM:** CrossFit **PM:** 4–5 × 400 m/ easy 400 m betw. each	CrossFit or OFF
	ELITE	CrossFit	**AM:** 20–30 min. drills 5–6 × 400 m/ rest 1:30 betw. each **PM:** CrossFit	**AM:** 20–30 min. drills 5 mi. @ 80% of 5K race pace **PM:** CrossFit or OFF
WEEK 3	BEGINNER	CrossFit	**AM:** 30–45 min. drills 4–5 × 400 m/ easy 400 m betw. each **PM:** CrossFit	CrossFit (run bias) or OFF
	INTERMEDIATE	CrossFit/CFE S & C Recovery*/OFF	**AM:** 20–30 min. drills 4–5 × 400 m/ easy 300 m betw. each **PM:** CrossFit	CrossFit (run bias) or OFF
	ELITE	CrossFit/CFE S & C Recovery/OFF	**AM:** 20–30 min. drills 5K @ 85% of 5K race pace w/3 × 400 m @ 110% of 5K race pace in middle of 5K/2–3 min. @ 5K race pace betw. each **PM:** CrossFit	CrossFit

T	F	S	S
45 min. drills 2–3 × 800 m/ rest 3:00 betw. each	CrossFit or OFF	CrossFit or OFF	30 min. drills 5K TT
30–45 min. drills 4–5 × 800 m/ rest 2:30 betw. each	CrossFit or OFF	30 min. drills 5K TT	CrossFit
20–30 min. drills 6–8 × 800 m/ rest 2:30 betw. each	CrossFit or OFF	**AM:** CrossFit or OFF **PM:** 15–20 min. drills 5K @ 80% of 5K race pace	15 min. drills 5K TT, same course as yesterday
45 min. drills 3 × 800 m/ rest 3:00 betw. each	CrossFit (run bias) or OFF	30 min. drills 4 mi. @ 80% of 10K race pace	CrossFit or OFF
30–45 min. drills 4–5 × 800 m/ rest 2:30 betw. each	CrossFit or OFF	15–20 min. drills 5K @ 80% of 5K TT pace	CrossFit (run bias)
20–30 min. drills 6–8 × 800 m/ easy 600 m betw. each	CrossFit or OFF	**AM:** 45 min. drills **PM:** CrossFit or OFF	15 min. drills 5 mi. @ 90% of 10K race pace
30–45 min. drills 3–4 × 800 m/ rest 2:45 betw. each	CrossFit or OFF	CrossFit or OFF	30 min. drills 4 mi. TT
30–45 min. drills 6–8 × 800 m/ rest 2:30 betw. each	CrossFit or OFF	15–20 min. drills 4 mi. TT	CrossFit (run bias) @ 80–90% effort or OFF
30–45 min. drills 6–8 × 800 m/ rest 2:00 betw. each	CrossFit (run bias) or OFF	15–20 min. drills 10K TT	**AM:** 30 min. drills 5K @ 80% of 10K race pace **PM:** CrossFit or OFF

CONTINUED

MARATHON TRAINING PLAN *continued*

	LEVEL	M	T	W
WEEK 4	**BEGINNER**	CrossFit/CFE S & C Recovery/OFF	**AM:** 30–45 min. drills 5+ × 400 m/ easy 300 m betw. each **PM:** CrossFit	CrossFit (run bias)
	INTERMEDIATE	CrossFit	**AM:** 20–30 min. drills 5+ × 400 m/ rest 1:30 betw. each **PM:** CrossFit	CrossFit
	ELITE	CrossFit/CFE S & C Recovery/OFF	**AM:** 20–30 min. drills 6–8 × 400 m/ easy 400 m betw. each **PM:** CrossFit	CrossFit
WEEK 5	**BEGINNER**	OFF	**AM:** 30–45 min. drills 5+ × 400 m/ rest 1:45 betw. each **PM:** CrossFit	CrossFit
	INTERMEDIATE	CrossFit/CFE S & C Recovery/OFF	**AM:** 20–30 min. drills 6+ × 400 m/ easy 300 m betw. each **PM:** CrossFit	CrossFit (run bias)
	ELITE	CrossFit/CFE S & C Recovery/OFF	**AM:** 20–30 min. drills 10K @ 85% of 10K race pace **PM:** CrossFit or OFF	CrossFit (run bias)
WEEK 6	**BEGINNER**	CrossFit	**AM:** 30–45 min. drills 5+ × 400 m/ easy 300 m betw. each **PM:** CrossFit	CrossFit
	INTERMEDIATE	CrossFit/CFE S & C Recovery/OFF	**AM:** 20–30 min. drills 5K @ 90% of 5K race pace **PM:** CrossFit	CrossFit
	ELITE	CrossFit/CFE S & C Recovery/OFF	**AM:** 20–30 min. drills 8+ × 400 m/ rest 1:30 betw. each **PM:** CrossFit	CrossFit (run bias)

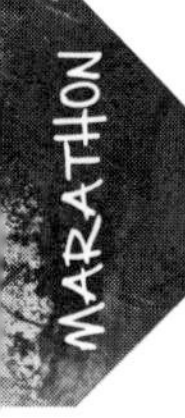

T	F	S	S
30–45 min. drills 4–5 × 800 m/ rest 2:45 betw. each	CrossFit or OFF	**AM:** 30 min. drills 5K @ 80% of 5K race pace **PM:** 15 min. drills 5K @ 85%+ of 5K race pace	CrossFit @ 80% effort or OFF
30–45 min. drills 3–4 × 1000 m/ easy 600 m betw. each	CrossFit (run bias) or OFF	**AM:** 30 min. drills Tabata sprints **PM:** CrossFit or OFF	15–20 min. drills 10K TT
30 min. drills 5 mi. @ 85% of 5K race pace	CrossFit or OFF	CrossFit	30 min. drills 3 × 5K @ 80%+ of 5K race pace, split morning, noon, evening
30–45 min. drills 4–5 × 800 m/ easy 400 m betw. each	CrossFit or OFF	CrossFit	20–30 min. drills 10K TT
30–45 min. drills 4–5 × 1000 m/ rest 3:00 betw. each	CrossFit	CrossFit or OFF	15–20 min. drills 10 mi. @ 80% of 10K TT pace
30–45 min. drills 5+ × 1000 m/ rest 2:30 betw. each	CrossFit	15–20 min. drills 4 × 1 mi. @ 5K race pace/ rest 3:00 betw. each	30 min. drills 10 mi. @ 85% of 10K race pace
30–45 min. drills 5–6 × 800 m/ rest 2:30 betw. each	CrossFit or OFF	30 min. drills 2 × 5K TT/ rest 10:00 betw.	CrossFit/CFE S & C Recovery/OFF
30–45 min. drills 4+ × 1000 m/ easy 600 m betw. each	CrossFit (run bias) or OFF	20–30 min. drills 10K @ 90% of 10K race pace	**AM:** 30 min. drills Tabata sprints **PM:** CrossFit or OFF
30–45 min. drills 10K @ 90% of 10K race pace	CrossFit	15–20 min. drills 15 mi. @ 80% of half-marathon race pace	**AM:** CFE S & C Recovery **PM:** 30 min. drills Tabata sprints

CONTINUED

MARATHON TRAINING PLAN *continued*

	LEVEL	M	T	W
WEEK 7	BEGINNER	CrossFit	**AM:** 30–45 min. drills 4 × 600 m/ easy 400 m betw. each **PM:** CrossFit	CrossFit
	INTERMEDIATE	CrossFit/CFE S & C Recovery/OFF	**AM:** 20–30 min. drills 6+ × 600 m/ easy 300 m betw. each **PM:** CrossFit	CrossFit (run bias)
	ELITE	CrossFit/CFE S & C Recovery/OFF	**AM:** 30 min. drills 6+ × 1000 m/ easy 500 m betw. each **PM:** CrossFit	CrossFit (run bias)
WEEK 8	BEGINNER	CrossFit	**AM:** 30–45 min. drills 5–6 × 600 m/ rest 2:00 betw. each **PM:** CrossFit	CrossFit (run bias)
	INTERMEDIATE	CrossFit/CFE S & C Recovery/OFF	**AM:** 20–30 min. drills 5 mi. @ 85% of 10K race pace	CrossFit (run bias)
	ELITE	CrossFit/CFE S & C Recovery/OFF	**AM:** 20 min. drills 10K @ 80% of 10K race pace **PM:** CrossFit	CrossFit (run bias)
WEEK 9	BEGINNER	CrossFit	**AM:** 30–45 min. drills 5–6 × 400 m/ easy 300 m betw. each **PM:** CrossFit	CrossFit (run bias)
	INTERMEDIATE	CrossFit/CFE S & C Recovery/OFF	**AM:** 20–30 min. drills 6+ × 400 m/ easy 300 m betw. each **PM:** CrossFit	CrossFit (run bias)
	ELITE	CrossFit/CFE S & C Recovery/OFF	**AM:** 20 min. drills 8+ × 400 m/ easy 300 m betw. each **PM:** CrossFit	CrossFit (run bias)

T	F	S	S
30–45 min. drills 3–4 × 1000 m/ rest 3:30 betw. each	CrossFit (run bias)	OFF	30 min. drills 15K at 80% of 10K race pace
30–45 min. drills 5+ × 1000 m/ rest 3:00 betw. each	CrossFit	20–30 min. drills 12 mi. @ 80% of half-marathon race pace	**AM:** 30 min. drills Tabata sprints **PM:** CrossFit or OFF
30 min. drills 7 mi. @ 80% of 10K race pace	**AM:** CrossFit **PM:** 15 min. drills Tabata sprints	15–20 min. drills 3 × 5 mi. @ 90%+ of 10K race pace split morning, noon, evening	**AM:** 30 min. drills Tabata sprints **PM:** CrossFit or OFF
30–45 min. drills 3–4 × 1000 m/ easy 600 m betw. each	CrossFit	OFF	30 min. drills 10 mi. TT
30–45 min. drills 5+ × 1000 m/ easy 500 m betw. each	**AM:** 30 min. drills Tabata sprints **PM:** CrossFit or OFF	CrossFit or OFF	15–20 min. drills 13.1 mi. TT
30–45 min. drills 6+ × 1000 m/ easy 500 m betw. each	**AM:** CrossFit **PM:** 15 min. drills Tabata sprints	15–20 min. drills 20 mi. @ 90%+ of marathon goal race pace	**AM:** CFE S & C Recovery **PM:** 30 min. drills 4 × 1 mi. @ 80% of 5K race pace/ rest 3:00 betw. each
30–45 min. drills 3–4 × 1000 m/ rest 3:00 betw. each	CrossFit	OFF	30 min. drills 12 mi. @ 80% of 10 mi. TT pace
15 min. drills 10K @ 80% of 10K race pace	**AM:** 30 min. drills Tabata sprints **PM:** CrossFit or OFF	CrossFit or OFF	**AM:** 15–20 min. drills 2 × 5K TT/ rest 10:00 betw. **PM:** 15–20 min. drills 2 × 5K @ 90% of AM pace/ rest 10:00 betw.
30–45 min. drills 6+ × 1000 m/ rest 2:30 betw. each	**AM:** CrossFit **PM:** 15 min. drills Tabata sprints	15–20 min. drills 5K @ 80%+ of 5K race pace	20–30 min. drills 13.1 mi. TT

CONTINUED

MARATHON TRAINING PLAN *continued*

	LEVEL	M	T	W
WEEK 10	BEGINNER	CrossFit	**AM:** 30–45 min. drills 5–6 × 600 m/ easy 300 m betw. each **PM:** CrossFit	CrossFit (run bias)
	INTERMEDIATE	CrossFit/CFE S & C Recovery/OFF	**AM:** 20–30 min. drills 6+ × 600 m/ easy 300 m betw. each **PM:** CrossFit	CrossFit (run bias)
	ELITE	CrossFit/CFE S & C Recovery/OFF	**AM:** 20 min. drills 10K @ 80% of 10K race pace **PM:** CrossFit or OFF	CrossFit (run bias)
WEEK 11	BEGINNER	CrossFit	**AM:** 30–45 min. drills 5–6 × 400 m/ easy 300 m betw. each **PM:** CrossFit	CrossFit (run bias)
	INTERMEDIATE	CrossFit/CFE S & C Recovery/OFF	**AM:** 20–30 min. drills 7 mi. @ 80–90% of 10K race pace	CrossFit (run bias)
	ELITE	CrossFit/CFE S & C Recovery/OFF	**AM:** 20 min. drills 10K @ 80% of 10K race pace **PM:** CrossFit or OFF	CrossFit (run bias)

T	F	S	S
30–45 min. drills 2 × 200 m/rest 1:30 + 2 × 400m/rest 1:30 + 2 × 1000 m/rest 3:00 betw. each	CrossFit or OFF	30 min. drills 13.1 mi. @ 90% of 12 mi. (last week)	CrossFit (run bias) or OFF
30–45 min. drills 2 × 200 m/rest 1:30 + 2 × 400 m/rest 1:30 + 3 × 1000 m/rest 3:00 betw. each	CrossFit (run bias) or OFF	15–20 min. drills 13.1 mi. @ 80% of half-marathon race pace	15–20 min. drills 2 × 5K @ 80–90% of 5K race pace/ rest 10:00 betw.
30–45 min. drills 3 × 200 m/rest 1:30 + 3 × 400 m/rest 1:30 + 4 × 1000 m/rest 3:00 betw. each	CrossFit (run bias) or OFF	15–20 min. drills 20 mi. @ 80% of 13.1 mi. TT pace	30 min. drills 2 × 5K @ 80%+ of 10K race pace/rest 5:00–10:00 betw.
30–45 min. drills 3 × 200 m/rest 1:30 + 3 × 400 m/rest 1:30 + 2 × 1000 m/rest 3:00 betw. each	CrossFit	OFF	30 min. drills 13.1 mi. TT
30–45 min. drills 4 × 200 m/rest 1:30 + 2 × 400 m/rest 1:30 + 3 × 1000 m/rest 3:00 betw. each	CrossFit (run bias) or OFF	15–20 min. drills 15 mi. @ 80% of 13.1 mi. TT pace	15–20 min. drills 3 × 5K @ 80–90% of 5K race pace
30–45 min. drills 3 × 200 m/rest 1:30 + 3 × 400 m/rest 1:30 + 4 × 1000 m/rest 3:00 betw. each	CrossFit (run bias) or OFF	15–20 min. drills 10 mi. @ 80% of 10 mi. TT pace	30 min. drills 10K @ 90%+ of 10K race pace

CONTINUED

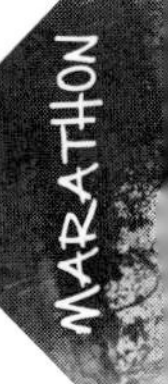

MARATHON TRAINING PLAN *continued*

	LEVEL	M	T	W
WEEK 12	BEGINNER	CFE S & C Recovery	**AM:** 30–45 min. drills 8 × 400 m/ easy 200 m betw. each **PM:** CrossFit or OFF	CrossFit (run bias) or OFF
WEEK 12	INTERMEDIATE	CrossFit/CFE S & C Recovery/OFF	**AM:** 20–30 min. drills 6+ × 600 m/ easy 400 m betw. each **PM:** CrossFit	CrossFit (run bias)
WEEK 12	ELITE	CrossFit/CFE S & C Recovery/OFF	30–45 min. drills 3 × 200 m/rest 1:30 + 3 × 400 m/rest 1:30 + 4 × 1000 m/rest 3:00 betw. each	CrossFit (run bias)
TAPER WEEK	ALL LEVELS	**AM:** Squat 5 × 3 or 5 × 5 at 80–90% of usual weight **PM:** 8–12 × 200 m/ rest 2:00 betw. each. Hold paces you held at start of program. Focus on technique.	Easy 30 min. run	Easy walking or OFF

200s: 98+ cadence **300s:** 98+ cadence **400s:** 98+ cadence **600s:** 98+ cadence **800s:** 96+ cadence
1000s: 95+ cadence **1200s:** 95+ cadence **1 mi.:** 95+ cadence **2 mi.:** 95+ cadence **5K:** 95+ cadence
You should be able to maintain the same relative pace for each of these intervals.

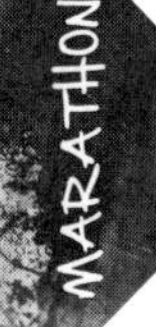

T	F	S	S
30–45 min. drills 4 × 200 m/rest 1:30 + 3 × 400 m/rest 1:30 + 2 × 1000 m/rest 3:00 betw. each	CrossFit (run bias)	**AM:** 30 min. drills 2 × 5K TT/ rest 10:00 betw. **PM:** 15–20 min. drills 2 × 5K TT/ rest 10:00 betw.	CFE S & C Recovery
30–45 min. drills 4 × 200 m/rest 1:30 + 3 × 400 m/rest 1:30 + 2 × 1000 m/rest 3:00 betw. each	CrossFit (run bias) or OFF	15–20 min. drills 18 mi. TT	**AM:** CFE S & C Recovery **PM:** 15 min. drills 2 × 5K @ 80% of 5K race pace/ rest 10:00 betw.
AM: 20 min. drills 10K @ 80% of 10K race pace **PM:** CrossFit or OFF	CrossFit (run bias) or OFF	15–20 min. drills 20 mi. TT	**AM:** CFE S & C Recovery **PM:** 15 min. drills 10K @ 80% of 10K race pace
AM: 3–5 RFT of 5 pull-ups, 10 push-ups, 15 squats **PM:** 3–4 × 400 m @ 70% effort, walk 200 m betw. each. Focus on technique.	Easy walking or OFF	RACE or easy 20–30 min. run	RACE + CFE S & C Recovery

+1/+2/+3, etc., simply means to continue until you are too fatigued for your technique and form to hold up.

**The CFE S & C recovery circuit may be found in Chapter 5, page 127.*

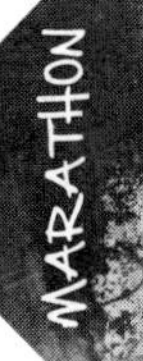

ULTRA TRAINING PLAN

	LEVEL	M	T	W
WEEK 1	BEGINNER	CrossFit	**AM:** 45 min. drills 6–8 × 200 m/ rest 2:00 betw. each **PM:** CrossFit	CrossFit (run bias) or OFF
	INTERMEDIATE	CrossFit	**AM:** 30–45 min. drills 8–10 × 200 m/ rest 2:00 betw. each **PM:** CrossFit	CrossFit (run bias) or OFF
	ELITE	CrossFit	**AM:** 20–30 min. drills 10–12 × 200 m/ rest 1:30 betw. each **PM:** CrossFit	20–30 min. drills 5K @ 85% of 10K race pace
WEEK 2	BEGINNER	CrossFit	**AM:** 30–45 min. drills 8–10 × 200 m/ easy 300 m betw. each **PM:** CrossFit	CrossFit or OFF
	INTERMEDIATE	5K @ 80% of 5K TT pace	**AM:** CrossFit **PM:** 4–5 × 400 m/ easy 400 m betw. each	CrossFit or OFF
	ELITE	CrossFit	**AM:** 20–30 min. drills 5–6 × 400 m/ easy 300 m betw. each **PM:** CrossFit	**AM:** 20–30 min. drills 5 mi. @ 80% of 5K race pace **PM:** CrossFit or OFF
WEEK 3	BEGINNER	CrossFit	**AM:** 30–45 min. drills 4–5 × 400 m/ easy 300 m betw. each **PM:** CrossFit	CrossFit (run bias) or OFF
	INTERMEDIATE	CrossFit/CFE S & C Recovery*/OFF	**AM:** 20–30 min. drills 4–5 × 400 m/ rest 1:30 betw. each **PM:** CrossFit	CrossFit (run bias) or OFF
	ELITE	CrossFit/CFE S & C Recovery/OFF	**AM:** 20–30 min. drills 5K @ 85% of 5K race pace w/3 × 400 m @ race pace in middle **PM:** CrossFit	CrossFit

T	F	S	S
45 min. drills 2–3 × 3:00/ rest 3:00 betw. each	CrossFit or OFF	CrossFit or OFF	30 min. drills 5K trail TT
30–45 min. drills 4–5 × 2:45/ rest 2:45 betw. each	CrossFit or OFF	30 min. drills 5K trail TT	CrossFit
20–30 min. drills 6–8 × 2:30/ rest 2:30 betw. each	CrossFit or OFF	**AM:** CrossFit or OFF **PM:** 15–20 min. drills 5K trail @ 80% of 5K race pace	15 min. drills 5K trail TT, same course as yesterday
45 min. drills 3 × 3:00/ rest 3:00 betw. each	CrossFit (run bias) or OFF	30 min. drills 5K trail @ 80% of 5K TT pace	CrossFit or OFF
30–45 min. drills 4–5 × 2:45/ rest 2:30 betw. each	CrossFit or OFF	15–20 min. drills 5 mi. trail @ 80% of 5K TT pace	CrossFit (run bias)
20–30 min. drills 6–8 × 2:30/ rest 2:30 betw. each	CrossFit or OFF	**AM:** 45 min. drills **PM:** CrossFit or OFF	15 min. drills 5 mi. trail @ 90% of 10K race pace
30–45 min. drills 3–4 × 3:00/ rest 2:45 betw. each	CrossFit or OFF	CrossFit or OFF	30 min. drills 10K trail TT
30–45 min. drills 6–8 × 2:45/ rest 2:30 betw. each	CrossFit or OFF	15–20 min. drills 10K trail TT	CrossFit (run bias) @ 80–90% effort or OFF
30–45 min. drills 6–8 × 2:30/ rest 2:00 betw. each	CrossFit (run bias) or OFF	15–20 min. drills 10K trail TT	**AM:** 30 min. drills 5K @ 80% of 10K race pace **PM:** CrossFit or OFF

CONTINUED

ULTRA TRAINING PLAN *continued*

	LEVEL	M	T	W
WEEK 4	BEGINNER	CrossFit/CFE S & C Recovery/OFF	**AM:** 30–45 min. drills 8 × 300 m/ easy 300 m betw. each **PM:** CrossFit	CrossFit (run bias)
	INTERMEDIATE	CrossFit	**AM:** 20–30 min. drills 5–6 × 400 m/ easy 300 m betw. each **PM:** CrossFit	CrossFit
	ELITE	CrossFit/CFE S & C Recovery/OFF	**AM:** 20–30 min. drills 6–8 × 400 m/ easy 400 m betw. each **PM:** CrossFit	CrossFit
WEEK 5	BEGINNER	OFF	**AM:** 30–45 min. drills 5–6 × 400 m/ easy 300 m betw. each **PM:** CrossFit	CrossFit
	INTERMEDIATE	CrossFit/CFE S & C Recovery/OFF	**AM:** 20–30 min. drills 6–8 × 400 m/ easy 300 m betw. each **PM:** CrossFit	CrossFit (run bias)
	ELITE	CrossFit/CFE S & C Recovery/OFF	**AM:** 20–30 min. drills 10K @ 85% of 10K race pace **PM:** CrossFit or OFF	CrossFit (run bias)
WEEK 6	BEGINNER	CrossFit	**AM:** 30–45 min. drills 5–6 × 400 m/ easy 300 m betw. each **PM:** CrossFit	CrossFit
	INTERMEDIATE	CrossFit/CFE S & C Recovery/OFF	**AM:** 20–30 min. drills 5K trail @ 90% of 5K race pace **PM:** CrossFit	CrossFit
	ELITE	CrossFit/CFE S & C Recovery/OFF	**AM:** 20–30 min. drills 8+ × 400 m/ easy 300 m betw. each **PM:** CrossFit	CrossFit (run bias)

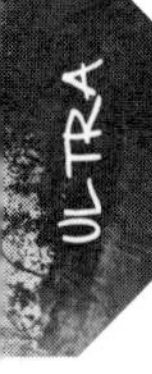

T	F	S	S
30–45 min. drills 4–5 × 3:00/ rest 2:45 betw. each	CrossFit or OFF	**AM:** 30 min. drills 5K trail @ 80% of 5K race pace **PM:** 15 min. drills 5K @ 85%+ of 5K race pace	CrossFit @ 80% effort or OFF
30–45 min. drills 3–4 × 3:45/ rest 3:00 betw. each	CrossFit (run bias) or OFF	**AM:** 30 min. drills Tabata sprints **PM:** CrossFit or OFF	15–20 min. drills 10K trail TT
30 min. drills 5 mi. trail @ 85% of 5K race pace	CrossFit or OFF	CrossFit	30 min. drills 3 × 5K trail @ 80%+ of 5K race pace split morning, noon, evening
30–45 min. drills 4–5 × 3:00/ rest 2:30 betw. each	CrossFit or OFF	CrossFit	20–30 min. drills 10K trail TT
30–45 min. drills 4–5 × 3:30/ rest 3:00 betw. each	CrossFit	CrossFit or OFF	15–20 min. drills 10 mi. trail @ 80% of 10K TT pace
30–45 min. drills 5+ × 3:00/ easy 2:30 betw. each	CrossFit	15–20 min. drills 4 × 1 mi. @ 5K race pace/ rest 3:00 betw. each	30 min. drills 10 mi. trail @ 85% of 10K race pace
30–45 min. drills 5–6 × 3:00/ rest 2:30 betw. each	CrossFit or OFF	30 min. drills 2 × 5K trail TT/ rest 10:00 betw.	CrossFit/CFE S & C Recovery/OFF
30–45 min. drills 4+ × 3:30/ rest 3:00 betw. each	CrossFit (run bias) or OFF	20–30 min. drills 10K trail @ 90% of 10K race pace	**AM:** 30 min. drills Tabata sprints **PM:** CrossFit or OFF
30–45 min. drills 10K trail @ 90% of 10K race pace	CrossFit	15–20 min. drills 15 mi. trail @ 80% of half-marathon race pace	**AM:** CFE S & C Recovery **PM:** 30 min. drills Tabata sprints

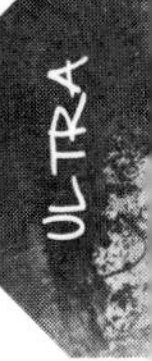

CONTINUED

ULTRA TRAINING PLAN *continued*

	LEVEL	M	T	W
WEEK 7	**BEGINNER**	CrossFit	**AM:** 30–45 min. drills 4 × 600 m/ rest 2:00 betw. each **PM:** CrossFit	CrossFit
	INTERMEDIATE	CrossFit/CFE S & C Recovery/OFF	**AM:** 20–30 min. drills 6+ × 600 m/ rest 1:30 betw. each **PM:** CrossFit	CrossFit (run bias)
	ELITE	CrossFit/CFE S & C Recovery/OFF	**AM:** 30 min. drills 6+ × 1000 m/ rest 2:30 betw. each **PM:** CrossFit	CrossFit (run bias)
WEEK 8	**BEGINNER**	CrossFit	**AM:** 30–45 min. drills 5–6 × 600 m/ easy 400 m betw. each **PM:** CrossFit	CrossFit (run bias)
	INTERMEDIATE	CrossFit/CFE S & C Recovery/OFF	**AM:** 20–30 min. drills 5 mi. trail @ 85% of 10K race pace	CrossFit (run bias)
	ELITE	CrossFit/CFE S & C Recovery/OFF	**AM:** 20 min. drills 10K trail @ 80% of 10K race pace **PM:** CrossFit	CrossFit (run bias)
WEEK 9	**BEGINNER**	CrossFit	**AM:** 30–45 min. drills 5–6 × 400 m/ easy 300 m betw. each **PM:** CrossFit	CrossFit (run bias)
	INTERMEDIATE	CrossFit/CFE S & C Recovery/OFF	**AM:** 20–30 min. drills 8+ × 400 m/ rest 1:30 betw. each **PM:** CrossFit	CrossFit (run bias)
	ELITE	CrossFit/CFE S & C Recovery/OFF	**AM:** 20 min. drills 8+ × 400 m/ easy 300 m betw. each **PM:** CrossFit	CrossFit (run bias)

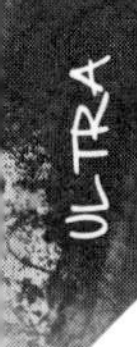

T	F	S	S
30–45 min. drills 3–4 × 4:00/ easy 3:30 betw. each	CrossFit (run bias)	OFF	30 min. drills 15K trail at 80% of 10K race pace
30–45 min. drills 5+ × 3:30/ rest 3:00 betw. each	CrossFit	20–30 min. drills 12 mi. trail @ 80% of half-marathon race pace	**AM:** 30 min. drills Tabata sprints **PM:** CrossFit or OFF
30 min. drills 7 mi. trail @ 80% of 10K race pace	**AM:** CrossFit **PM:** 15 min. drills Tabata sprints	15–20 min. drills 3 × 5 mi. trail @ 90%+ of 10K race pace split morning, noon, evening	**AM:** 30 min. drills Tabata sprints **PM:** CrossFit or OFF
30–45 min. drills 3–4 × 4:00/ rest 3:00 betw. each	CrossFit	OFF	30 min. drills 10 mi. trail TT
30–45 min. drills 5+ × 3:30/ rest 2:30 betw. each	**AM:** 30 min. drills Tabata sprints **PM:** CrossFit or OFF	CrossFit or OFF	15–20 min. drills 13.1 mi. trail TT
30–45 min. drills 6+ × 1000 m/ rest 2:30 betw. each	**AM:** CrossFit **PM:** 15 min. drills Tabata sprints	15–20 min. drills 20 mi. trail @ 90%+ of 50K race pace	**AM:** CFE S & C Recovery **PM:** 30 min. drills 4 × 1 mi. @ 80% of 5K race pace/ rest 3:00 betw. each
30–45 min. drills 3–4 × 4:00/ rest 3:00 betw. each	CrossFit	OFF	30 min. drills 12 mi. trail @ 80% of 10 mi. TT pace
15 min. drills 10K trail @ 80% of 10K race pace	**AM:** 30 min. drills Tabata sprints **PM:** CrossFit or OFF	CrossFit or OFF	**AM:** 15–20 min. drills 2 × 5K trail TT/ rest 10:00 betw. **PM:** 15–20 min. drills 2 × 5K @ 90% of AM/rest 10:00 betw.
30–45 min. drills 6+ × 3:00/ rest 2:30 betw. each	**AM:** CrossFit **PM:** 15 min. drills Tabata sprints	15–20 min. drills 5K @ 80%+ of 5K race pace	20–30 min. drills 13.1 mi. trail TT

ULTRA

CONTINUED

ULTRA TRAINING PLAN *continued*

	LEVEL	M	T	W
WEEK 10	BEGINNER	CrossFit	**AM:** 30–45 min. drills 5–6 × 2:00/ rest 1:30 betw. each **PM:** CrossFit	CrossFit (run bias)
	INTERMEDIATE	CrossFit/CFE S & C Recovery/OFF	**AM:** 20–30 min. drills 6+ × 1:45/ easy 300 m betw. each **PM:** CrossFit	CrossFit (run bias)
	ELITE	CrossFit/CFE S & C Recovery/OFF	**AM:** 20 min. drills 10K trail @ 80% of 10K race pace **PM:** CrossFit or OFF	CrossFit (run bias)
WEEK 11	BEGINNER	CrossFit	**AM:** 30–45 min. drills 5–6 × 1:30/ easy 300 m betw. each **PM:** CrossFit	CrossFit (run bias)
	INTERMEDIATE	CrossFit/CFE S & C Recovery/OFF	**AM:** 20–30 min. drills 7 mi. trail @ 80–90% of 10K race pace	CrossFit (run bias)
	ELITE	CrossFit/CFE S & C Recovery/OFF	**AM:** 20 min. drills 10K trail @ 80% of 10K race pace **PM:** CrossFit or OFF	CrossFit (run bias)

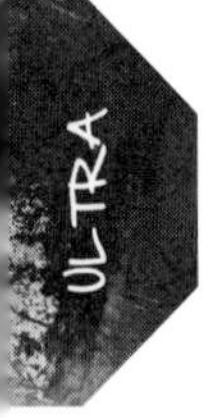

T	F	S	S
30–45 min. drills 2 × 200 m/rest 1:30 + 2 × 400 m/rest 1:30 + 2 × 1000 m/rest 3:00 betw. each	CrossFit or OFF	30 min. drills 13.1 mi. trail @ 90% of 12 mi. (last week)	CrossFit (run bias) or OFF
30–45 min. drills 2 × 200 m/rest 1:30 + 2 × 400 m/rest 1:30 + 3 × 1000 m/rest 3:00 betw. each	CrossFit (run bias) or OFF	15–20 min. drills 13.1 mi. trail @ 80% of half-marathon race pace	15–20 min. drills 2 × 5K @ 80–90% of 5K race pace/ rest 10:00 betw.
30–45 min. drills 3 × 200 m/rest 1:30 + 3 × 400 m/rest 1:30 + 4 × 1000 m/rest 3:00 betw. each	CrossFit (run bias) or OFF	15–20 min. drills 20 mi. trail @ 80% of 13.1 mi. TT pace	30 min. drills 2 × 5K @ 80%+ of 10K race pace/rest 5:00–10:00 betw.
30–45 min. drills 3 × 200 m/rest 1:30 + 3 × 400 m/rest 1:30 + 2 × 1000 m/rest 3:00 betw. each	CrossFit	OFF	30 min. drills 13.1 mi. trail TT
30–45 min. drills 4 × 200 m/rest 1:30 + 2 × 400 m/rest 1:30 + 3 × 1000 m/rest 3:00 betw. each	CrossFit (run bias) or OFF	15–20 min. drills 15 mi. trail @ 80% of 13.1 mi. TT pace	15–20 min. drills 3 × 5K @ 80–90% of 5K race pace
30–45 min. drills 3 × 200 m/rest 1:30 + 3 × 400 m/rest 1:30 + 4 × 1000 m/rest 3:00 betw. each	CrossFit (run bias) or OFF	15–20 min. drills 10 mi. trail @ 80% of 10 mi. TT pace	30 min. drills 10K trail @ 90%+ of 10K race pace

CONTINUED

ULTRA TRAINING PLAN *continued*

	LEVEL	M	T	W
WEEK 12	**BEGINNER**	CFE S & C Recovery	**AM:** 30–45 min. drills 8 × 1:30/ easy 1:15 betw. each **PM:** CrossFit or OFF	CrossFit (run bias) or OFF
	INTERMEDIATE	CrossFit/CFE S & C Recovery/OFF	**AM:** 20–30 min. drills 6+ × 1:45/ easy 2:00 betw. each **PM:** CrossFit	CrossFit (run bias)
	ELITE	CrossFit/CFE S & C Recovery/OFF	30–45 min. drills 3 × 200 m/rest 1:30 + 3 × 400 m/rest 1:30 + 4 × 1000 m/rest 3:00 betw. each	CrossFit (run bias)
TAPER WEEK	**ALL LEVELS**	**AM:** Squat 5 × 3 or 5 × 5 at 80–90% of usual weight **PM:** 8–12 × 200 m/ rest 2:00 betw. each. Hold paces you held at start of program. Focus on technique.	Easy 30 min. run	Easy walking or OFF

200s: 98+ cadence **300s:** 98+ cadence **400s:** 98+ cadence **600s:** 98+ cadence **800s:** 96+ cadence
1000s: 95+ cadence **1200s:** 95+ cadence **1 mi.:** 95+ cadence **2 mi.:** 95+ cadence **5K:** 95+ cadence
You should be able to maintain the same relative pace for each of these intervals.

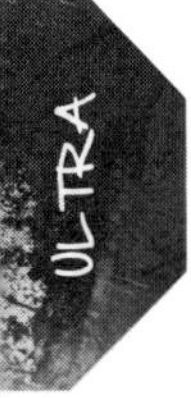

T	F	S	S
30–45 min. drills 4 × 200 m/rest 1:30 + 3 × 400 m/rest 1:30 + 2 × 1000 m/rest 3:00 betw. each	CrossFit (run bias)	**AM:** 30 min. drills 2 × 5K trail TT/ rest 10:00 betw. **PM:** 15–20 min. drills 2 × 5K trail TT/ rest 10:00 betw.	CFE S & C Recovery
30–45 min. drills 4 × 200 m/rest 1:30 + 3 × 400 m/rest 1:30 + 2 × 1000 m/rest 3:00 betw. each	CrossFit (run bias) or OFF	15–20 min. drills 18 mi. trail TT	**AM:** CFE S & C Recovery **PM:** 15 min. drills 2 × 5K trail @ 80% of 5K race pace/ rest 10:00 betw.
AM: 20 min. drills 10K trail @ 80% of 10K race pace **PM:** CrossFit or OFF	CrossFit (run bias) or OFF	15–20 min. drills 20 mi. trail TT	**AM:** CFE S & C Recovery **PM:** 15 min. drills 10K trail @ 80% of 10K race pace
AM: 3–5 RFT of 5 pull-ups, 10 push-ups, 15 squats **PM:** 3–4 × 400 m @ 70% effort, walk 200 m betw. each. Focus on technique.	Easy walking or OFF	RACE or easy 20–30 min. run	RACE + CFE S & C Recovery

+1/+2/+3, etc., simply means to continue until you are too fatigued for your technique and form to hold up.
Time-based intervals should be done on the same kind of terrain on which the athlete is racing.
**The CFE S & C recovery circuit may be found in Chapter 5, page 127.*

ULTRA

APPENDIX A
BUILDING YOUR HOME GYM

BARE-BONES HOME GYM

You can start building your home gym with just a kettlebell, a jump rope, and a place to install a pull-up bar. This will suffice for the many CFE workouts that use body weight only. At some point, however, you will want free weights. Although it is possible to do CrossFit workouts at fitness centers and commercial gyms, they generally don't have bumper plates (a necessity with Olympic lifts—dropping the barbells is routine when you pursue heavier lifts). Also, it can be tricky to do rounds of combinations of exercises in commercial gyms, since pairing pieces of equipment is challenging. Ultimately, joining a CrossFit gym or building your own gym complete with weights makes life easier.

GETTING STARTED

If you're just getting started and have space or budget restrictions, keep in mind that military units deployed to the field have designed effective CrossFit workouts using nothing more than a sandbag and other available equipment. And there is a group called the Fit for Life

Crew in Marion, Ohio, doing CrossFit in prison (part of an NAACP program) with nothing more than a jump rope and a room to train in. In other words, no excuses.

Here's a starter CrossFit gym you can throw into the trunk of your car and take to the park—ideally near a pull-up bar—for an outdoor workout:

- Jump rope
- Kettlebell or dumbbell
- Slam ball
- Medicine ball* for wall balls (do them against a basketball backboard or handball court)
- Sandbag for squats and Olympic lifts (buy a sandbag at a hardware store for pocket change; a 60-lb. bag should run you just a few dollars)
- Ab mat

THE IDEAL GARAGE GYM FOR A CFE ATHLETE

- Squat rack
- Barbell
- Barbell collars

---

* You can make a medicine ball with a used basketball, sand, and Gorilla Glue. Use pliers to take out the rubber plug in the ball, then pour sand into the ball using a funnel. Use Gorilla Glue to glue the plug back into the ball. Let it dry, then glue it up some more.

- 3 kettlebells: 35 lb., 53 lb., 72 lb. (kettlebells are pricey, so consider starting with a 35-lb. bell and collecting others as you progress)
- Bumper plates: 45 lb. × 6, 35 lb. × 2, 25 lb. × 2, 10 lb. × 2, 5 lb. × 2, 2.5 lb. × 2 (bumper plates are barbell weights with foam-rubber padding so they can be safely dropped to the ground—a must for Olympic lifting and working toward PRs in your powerlifting movements)
- Ab mat (a protective cushion for the lower back while doing sit-ups)
- Padded medicine ball: 20 lb. (for wall balls)
- Slam ball–style medicine ball: 40 lb. (for ball slams)
- Mobility bands: 4 strengths; used for pre- and postworkout mobility exercises
- Pull-up bar (anchor into the ceiling or a beam at a height you can reach safely)
- Plyometric box for box jumps (an 18- or 20-inch box is a good place to start)
- Jump rope

Great to have when you can afford it:

- Glute ham developer
- Rubber mats
- Dumbbells: 35 to 50 lb.
- Rowing ergometer

PLACES TO BUY EQUIPMENT

Squat racks, barbells, and weight equipment are available at most major sporting good stores, although selections of bumper plates and kettlebells can be harder to find. Jump ropes are easy to obtain. The most complete selections of CrossFit-specific equipment are currently found online. Here are several places to check out:

- Rogue (www.roguefitness.com)
- Again Faster (www.againfaster.com)
- Muscle Driver (www.MuscleDriverUSA.com)
- EliteFTS (www.elitefts.com)

APPENDIX B
ADVANCED INDIVIDUALIZED PROGRAMMING SAMPLE OF CFE

This appendix showcases how a CFE program can be tailored to the specific needs of an athlete. Using survey information, video analysis, and initial data captured in various strength, mobility, and endurance tests, Brian MacKenzie and Cody Burkhart created a training plan for an athlete that was based on his or her experience, strengths, and weaknesses.

A longtime associate of MacKenzie, Burkhart is a senior CFE coach and co-owner of an online athletic programming service, Athlete's Cell. He is an expert in mechanical and aerospace engineering (he also works for NASA's robotics division) and owner/coach at 1884 CrossFit in Denver, Colorado.

The following is a two-week sample from the program.

The language and notation used in the program will be easily understood by CrossFit coaches and those who have trained in a CrossFit environment for some time. However, for those new to CrossFit, some of this material will be unclear. To learn more, and to see the entire four-week training phase with videos of each of the movements mentioned—plus an explanatory interview—visit the web site unbreakablerunner.com.

Individualized CFE Sample, Week 1

	M	T	W
ACTIVATION	3 min. run (ham pull focus) or row (strapless w/glute focus) 5 × 10/10" OHS (10s down/10s up) 5 × 10/10" bench press 5 × 10/10" FS Perform with either PVC	3 min. row (focus on pull positioning of chest to floor angle maintenance) 5 × 10/10" muscle squat snatches Perform with either PVC	3 min. run (ham pull focus) 5 × 10/10" squat cleans Perform with either PVC 20 split jerk footwork drills
SKILL WORK	10 × skin the cats	20 × handstand shoulder touches	Barbell squat complex (empty bar) 3 × (5 BS, 5 FS, 5 OHS)
STRENGTH	CrossFit total #2: 3 × 1 OHS, 3 × 1 bench press, 3 × 1 clean REC. WORKING EACH LIFT AS 5-5-3-3-1-1-1	5 min. going over snatch lift technique 1 × Burgener warm-up (65/45), snatch focus Snatch to max in 15 min.	5 min. going over c&j lift technique 1 × Burgener warm-up (65/45), clean focus Clean and jerk to max in 15 min.
WOD	**OFF**	Diane (LVL 1) 21-15-9 DL (165/115) HSPU (MOD w/bands or box, NOT with stacked abmats)	10 min. EMOM 3 pull-ups 3HRPU + headstand to HSPU combos (switch to 3 HRPU SEPARATE from strict HSPU and then kipping as needed) 3 KB goblet squats (53/35) Drop to 2s if minute cannot be completed.

T	F	S	S
OFF	3 min. run (ham pull focus) or row (strapless w/glute focus) 5 × 10/10" DL (10s down/10s up) 5 × 10/10" strict press 5 × 10/10" BS Perform with either PVC	10 min. run @ 92 cadence	OFF
OFF	6 min. work up to max height box jump	10:00 CFE skills & drills Row or run based on WOD choice for athletes	OFF
OFF	CrossFit total: 3 × 1 back squat, 3 × 1 shoulder press, 3 × 1 deadlift REC. WORKING EACH LIFT AS 5-5-3-3-1-1-1	OFF	OFF
OFF	OFF	Roided-out Jackie (LVL 1) 2K row or run 50 thrusters (65/45) 10 C2B 10 chin-ups 10 pull-ups	OFF

CONTINUED

CONTINUED

Individualized CFE Sample, Week 1

	M	T	W
COOL-DOWN	3 min. row cooldown	3 min. row or Airdyne cooldown	3 min. run cooldown
RECOVERY	Quad mash + IT band lengthening	Snatch grip arch OH w/peanut mash	Banded distraction hip opener

T	F	S	S
OFF	5 min. row cooldown (strapless)	10 min. KB slow walk w/farmer's walk position (2 × 26/18) As few breaks as possible. Each time you break, perform 5 full sit-ups (no abmat).	OFF
OFF	5–10 min. squat test	30–60 min. mash session	OFF

Individualized CFE Sample, Week 2

	M	T	W
ACTIVATION	3 min. row (glute engagement focus) 5 × 10/10" DL (10s down/10s up) w/PVC 5 × 10/10" push-up 10 × cobra-style, straight-leg burpee to bwd roll to candlestick (bwd roll to candlestick to teach athlete to pull hands from ground to reduce torque loading)	3 min. run (ham pull focus) 5 × 10/10" snatch high pull 5 × 10/10" OHS 5 × 10/10" wall ball technique w/WB but no shot, just to full extension and back down	3 min. row (glute engagement focus) 5 × 10/10" power cleans 5 × 10/10" FS 10 × depth jumps (30/24) To perform depth jumps, athlete stands on box, steps off box, lands with both feet at same time, and attempts to jump as high as possible upon hitting the ground.
SKILL WORK	5 min. HSW skill work 5 min. PVC parallette skill work if enough equipment	1 × Burgener warm-up (PVC, 45/35), snatch focus 5 min. covering snatch complex	3 × 5 KB weighted depth jumps w/weight drop Athlete picks weight. Goal is to pick weight that does not engage golgi tendon reflex (i.e., a weight that does not turn off calf muscle and heel cord reaction and thus eliminate rebound ability). See video, but do not jump onto another box; just jump vertically as high as possible. www.youtube.com/watch?v=EMeRYuVoSgc
STRENGTH	WARM UP TO LOADS LISTED BELOW, then 6 min. ping-pong (On 3-2-1-GO complete your first set of 3, rest the remaining time in minute 1, then complete your first set of 7 in minute 2, rest the remainder of the time. Ping-pong back and forth until you complete all 5 sets of both movements.) 3 × 3 deadlift (75–85%) 3 × 7 OHS (65–70%)	**Part A:** Snatch to max in 10 min. (this is a daily max and does not need to be a lifetime PR, just how you feel that day). Then take 85% of your 1RPM for the day and complete 2 × 3 from the low hang position. **Part B:** Complete 3 sets of the following complex: 1 × clean, 1 × low hang clean and jerk, 1 × jerk (do not drop the bar during the complex)	5 min. warm-up BS and PP 6 min. ping-pong 3 × 3 back squat (75–85%) 3 × 7 push press (65–70%)

T	F	S	S
OFF	3 min. row (glute engagement focus) 5 × 10/10" FS 5 × 5" pistols 20 banded MU hip pop drills	1 mi. run @ 92 cadence	**OFF**
OFF	3 × 3 front lever (from inverted lower to ground as slow as possible, kip back to inverted) 3 × 3 back lever (from inverted lower to ground as slow as possible, kip back to inverted) Less experienced athletes use bands on low rings.	10 min. athlete choice	**OFF**
OFF	**Part A:** Clean and jerk to max in 10 min. (this is a daily max and does not need to be a lifetime PR, just how you feel that day). Then take 85% of your 1RPM for the day and complete 2 × 3 from the low hang position. **Part B:** Complete 3 sets of the following complex: 1 × snatch, 2 × low hang snatch (do not drop the bar during the complex)	5 min. warm-up thruster and PJ 6 min. ping-pong 3 × 3 thruster (75–80%) 3 × 7 push jerk (65–70%)	**OFF**

CONTINUED

CONTINUED

Individualized CFE Sample, Week 2

	M	T	W
WOD	10-1/1-10 DL (135/85) burpees 30 OHS (65/45)	16 min. EMOtherM **Even:** 1 snatch complex (1 PS + 1 SS + 3 OHS) weight of your choice May not release bar. If athlete cannot complete a full complex before minute is over, they must drop weight. **Odd:** Max SU to WB (14/10) Score is final weight of barbell + # of SU to WB	30 clean & jerks (75/55) 400 m run 15 burpee plate jumps (2 × 45/25)
COOLDOWN	3 min. row cooldown (strapless)	3 min. run or Airdyne cooldown	3 min. run cooldown
RECOVERY	Pec release w/lax ball against wall	Couch stretch	Wrist mobility work; see link: www.catalystathletics.com/media/video/video.php?videoID=114

T	F	S	S
OFF	10 min. EMOM 3 FS (95/65) 4 alt. pistols (use box sit method or hold plate in hands to offset CG) 4 MU transitions on low rings	BULL (LVL 1) 2RDS: 200 singles 30 pull-ups Run 1 mi. (35 min. cap)	OFF
OFF	3 min. row or Airdyne cooldown	10 min. KB slow walk w/ front rack walk position (2 × 26/18) As few breaks as possible. Each time you break, perform 5 TTR.	OFF
OFF	IT band lengthening	30–60 min. mash party	OFF

NOTES

INTRODUCTION

1. The term "functional" refers to compound exercise movements that recruit muscles throughout the body to produce work. Throwing a bale of hay, for example, is a functional movement. In CrossFit Endurance, functional, compound movements—such as a deadlift—are preferred over an exercise such as an arm curl, which isolates a single muscle.

2. VO_2max is a measurement of how efficiently a test subject processes oxygen; it is commonly used as a measurement of aerobic fitness.

3. I. Tabata, K. Nishimura, M. Kouzaki, Y. Hirai, F. Ogita, M. Miyachi, and K. Yamamoto, "Effects of Moderate-Intensity Endurance and High-Intensity Intermittent Training on Anaerobic Capacity and VO_2max," *Medicine and Science in Sports and Exercise* 28, 10 (1996): 1327–1330, doi:10.1097/00005768-199610000-00018, PMID 8897392.

4. M. J. Gibala, J. P. Little, M. van Essen, G. P. Wilkin, K. A. Burgomaster, A. Safdar, S. Raha, and M. A. Tarnopolsky, "Short-Term Sprint Interval Versus Traditional Endurance Training: Similar Initial Adaptations in Human Skeletal Muscle and Exercise Performance," *Journal of Physiology* 575 (2006): 901–911. See also Jonathan P. Little, Adeel S. Safdar, Geoffrey P. Wilkin, Mark A. Tarnopolsky, and Martin J. Gibala, "A Practical Model of Low-Volume High-Intensity Interval Training Induces Mitochondrial Biogenesis in Human Skeletal Muscle: Potential Mechanisms," *Journal of Physiology* 588 (2010): 1011–1022, doi:10.1113/jphysiol.2009.181743, PMC 2849965, PMID 20100740.

5. Adam Daoud, Gary Geissler, Frank Wang, Jason Saretsky, Yahya Daoud, and Daniel Lieberman, "Foot Strike and Injury Rates in Endurance Runners: A Retrospective Study," *Medicine and Science in Sports and Exercise* 44, 7 (2012): 1325–1334.

6. *2013 SFIA Sports, Fitness and Leisure Activities Topline Participation Report* (Sports and Fitness Industry Association, 2013).

CHAPTER 1: INDESTRUCTIBLE RUNNING FORM

1. Christopher McDougall, *Born to Run: A Hidden Tribe, Superathletes, and the Greatest Race the World Has Never Seen* (Random House, 2011).

2. Sara Germano, "The Five Fingers Question: Is Barefoot Running Any Good?" *Wall Street Journal*, May 8, 2014.

3. Ken Doherty, *Track and Field Omnibook* (Tafnews Press, 1971).

4. Nicholas Romanov, "Running Q&A and Debate—Romanov Versus McGee," USAT Art and Science of Triathlon Lecture Series, 2008.

5. Jennifer Kahn, "The Perfect Stride: Can Alberto Salazar Straighten Out American Distance Running?," *New Yorker*, November 8, 2010.

6. Adam I. Daoud, Gary J. Geissler, Frank Wang, Jason Saretsky, Yahya A. Daoud, and Daniel E. Lieberman, "Foot Strike and Injury Rates in Runners: A Retrospective Study," *Medicine and Science in Sports and Exercise* 44, 7 (2012): 1325–1334, doi: 10.1249/MSS.0b013e3182465115.

7. Larry Myers, *Training with Cerutty* (Anderson World, 1978).

8. Kelly Starrett, *Becoming a Supple Leopard: The Ultimate Guide to Resolving Pain, Preventing Injury, and Optimizing Athletic Performance* (Victory Belt, 2013).

9. Jay Dicharry, *Anatomy for Runners: Unlocking Your Athletic Potential for Health, Speed, and Injury Prevention* (Skyhorse Publishing, 2012).

10. Lyn Kukral, "Using Foot Shape to Select Running Shoe Is a 'Sports Myth,'" Army News Service, July 26, 2010..

CHAPTER 2: ENDURANCE WITH TEETH

1. M. Fredericson and A. K. Misra, "Epidemiology and Aetiology of Marathon Running Injuries," *Sports Medicine* 37 (2007): 437–439.

2. Owen Anderson, *Running Science* (Human Kinetics, 2013), 248–249.

3. S. L. Manske, C. R. Lorincz, and R. F. Zernicke, "Bone Health: Part 2, Physical Activity," *Sports Health: A Multidisciplinary Approach* 1 (2009): 341–346.

4. Tudor Bompa, PhD, and Michael C. Carrera, *Periodization Training for Sports* (Human Kinetics, 2005).

5. J. Jensen, J. Bangsbo, and Y. Hellsten, "Effect of High Intensity Training on Capillarization and Presence of Angiogenic Factors in Human Skeletal Muscle," *Journal of Applied Physiology* 557 (2004): 571–582.

6. A. Trembly, J. A. Simoneau, and C. Bouchard, "Impact of Exercise Intensity on Body Fatness and Skeletal Muscle Metabolism," *Metabolism* 43, 7 (1994): 814–818.

7. V. L. Billat, B. Elechet, B. Petit, G. Muriaux, and J. P. Koralsztein, "Interval Training at VO_2max: Effects on Aerobic Performance and Overtraining Markers," *Medicine and Science in Sports and Exercise* 31, 1 (1999): 156–163.

8. K. Burgomaster, S. Hughes, G. Heigenhauser, S. Bradwell, and M. Gibala, "Six Sessions of Sprint Interval Training Increases Muscle Oxidative Potential and Cycle Endurance Capacity in Humans," *Journal of Applied Physiology* 98, 6 (2005): 1985–1990.

9. Ed Coyle, "Very Intense Exercise Is Extremely Potent and Time Efficient: A Reminder," *Journal of Applied Physiology* 98, 6 (2005): 1983–1984.

10. L. Paavolainen, K. Häkinen, I. Hämälinen, A. Nummela, and H. Rusko, "Explosive Strength Training Improves 5K Running Time by Improving Running Economy and Muscle Power," *Journal of Applied Physiology* 86, 5 (1999): 1527–1533.

11. Anderson, *Running Science*.

12. Tim Noakes, *Lore of Running*, 4th ed. (Human Kinetics, 2002).

13. L. Nybo, "Hyperthermia and Fatigue," *Journal of Applied Physiology* 104, 3 (2008): 871–878.

CHAPTER 3: STRENGTH AND CONDITIONING WORKOUTS FOR THE CFE RUNNER

1. Functional exercises are compound in nature, recruiting an assortment of muscles throughout the body in patterns that occur in real-world situations. A tree falls on your friend, and you lift it off—you just used a functional movement. In contrast, if you use a Nautilus machine to train your trapezius muscles, that's an isolated exercise movement that trains one muscle and does not use a natural pattern.

2. R. N. van Gent, D. Siem, M. van Middelkoop, A. G. van Os, M. A. Bierma-Zeinstra, and B. W. Koes, "Incidence and Determinants of Lower Extremity Running Injuries in Long Distance Runners: A Systematic Review," *British Journal of Sports Medicine* 41, 8 (2007): 469–480.

3. Phil Latter, "Rethinking Running Health: Why Getting Injured Is a Frame of Mind," *Running Times*, March 2013.

4. R. C. Hickson, M. A. Rosenkoetter, and M. M. Brown, "Strength Training Effects on Aerobic Power and Short-Term Endurance," *Medicine and Science in Sports and Exercise* 12, 5 (1980): 336–339.

5. R. E. Johnston, T. J. Quinn, R. Kertzer, and N. Vroman, "Strength Training in Female Distance Runners: Impact on Running Economy," *Journal of Strength and Conditioning Research* 11, 4 (1997): 224–229.

6. L. Paavolainen, K. Häkkinen, I. Hämäläinen, A. Nummela, and H. Rusko, "Explosive-Strength Training Improves Running Economy and Muscle Power," *Journal of Applied Physiology* 86 (1999): 1527–1533.

7. Owen Anderson, *Running Science* (Human Kinetics, 2013), 136.

8. J. H. Wilmore, R. B. Parr, P. Ward, P. A. Vodak, T. J. Barstow, T. V. Pipes, G. Grimditch, and P. Leslie, "Energy Cost of Circuit Weight Training," *Medicine and Science in Sports* 10, 2 (1978): 75–78.

9. G. Klika and C. Jordan, "High-Intensity Circuit Training Using Bodyweight: Maximum Results with Minimum Investment," *ASCM Health and Fitness Journal* 17, 3 (2013): 8–13.

10. Ibid., 8.

11. "Anaerobic threshold" is a somewhat controversial term in the running world. In general, it refers to the speed a runner can hold at the point where lactic acid cannot be cleared from the muscles and begins to pool. The higher the threshold or lactate turning point, the more speed a runner can hold for a longer period of time.

CHAPTER 4: NUTRITION THE CROSSFIT ENDURANCE WAY

1. Kevin Helliker, "Why Runners Can't Eat Whatever They Want," *Wall Street Journal*, March 26, 2014.

2. Robert S. Schwartz, Stacia Merkel Kraus, Jonathan G. Schwartz, Kelly K. Wickstrom, Gretchen Peichel, Ross F. Garberich, John R. Lesser, Stephen N. Oesterle, Thomas Knickelbine, Kevin M. Harris, Sue Duval, William O. Roberts, and James H. O'Keefe, MD, "Increased Coronary Artery Plaque Volume Among Male Marathon Runners," *Missouri Medicine* 11 (2014): 85–90.

3. Matt Fitzgerald, "Should All Runners Now Eat McDonald's All the Time?," competitor.com, March 11, 2011.

4. K. Van Proeyen, K. Szlufckik, H. Nielsens, M. Ramaekers, and P. Hespel, "Beneficial Metabolic Adaptations Due to Endurance Exercise Training in the Fasted State," *Journal of Applied Physiology* 110, 1 (2011): 236–245.

5. Jeff Volek and Stephen Phinney, *The Art and Science of Low Carbohydrate Performance* (Beyond Obesity, 2012).

6. Tara P. Pope, "Switching to Grass-Fed Beef," http://well.blogs.nytimes.com/2010/03/11/switching-to-grass-fed-beef, March 11, 2010.

7. "Farmed Salmon and Human Health," Pure Salmon Campaign: Raising the Standards for Farm-Raised Fish, www.puresalmon.org/pdfs/human_health.pdf.

8. A. Shimotoyodome, J. Suzuki, Y. Kameo, and T. Hase, "Dietary Supplementation with Hydroxypropyl-Distarch Phosphate from Waxy Maize Starch Increases Resting Energy Expenditure by Lowering the Postprandial Glucose-Dependent Insulinotropic Polypeptide Response in Human Subjects," *British Journal of Nutrition* 6, 1 (2011): 96–104.

FURTHER READING

Astrand, Per-Olaf, Kaare Rodahl, Hans A. Dahl, and **Sigmund B. Stromme**. *Textbook of Work Physiology: Physiological Bases of Exercise,* 4th ed. Human Kinetics, 2003.

Lifting a rock off the ground, pulling yourself over a fence, or running down a road is more complex than you may think. This book explores the science and mechanics involved when the human body goes about getting physical work done.

Cavanagh, Peter, ed. *Biomechanics of Distance Running.* Human Kinetics, 1997.

A thorough dissection of the physics of distance running.

Coyle, Daniel. *The Talent Code: Greatness Isn't Born. It's Grown. Here's How.* Bantam, 2009.

Coyle explains the neuroscience involved in learning a new skill and showcases real-life stories that demonstrate how proper skill-building practices can produce stunning results.

Durant, John. *The Paleo Manifesto: Ancient Wisdom for Lifelong Health.* Harmony, 2014.

Durant examines the diet and habits cultivated by modern civilization and details how they are at odds with the way we are hardwired by evolution. He argues that this disconnect has resulted in chronic disease and dysfunction.

Lipton, Dr. Bruce. *The Biology of Belief: Unleashing the Power of Consciousness, Matter, and Miracles*, rev. ed. Hay House, 2013.

An advanced look at what science suggests is going on in the connection between thinking and reality, and how thought can directly impact the ways in which our genes are expressed.

MacKenzie, Brian, with **Glen Cordoza**. *Power, Speed, ENDURANCE: A Skill-Based Approach to Endurance Training*. Victory Belt Publishing, 2012.

A complete textbook covering MacKenzie's philosophy of making the skill of moving properly the number-one priority in an athlete's approach to running, swimming, and cycling. Provides detailed instructions and photos to guide readers through overhauling their form in each discipline. Also included are training protocols for strength, conditioning, and mobility and a template for creating your own CFE-type program.

Murphy, Michael. *The Future of the Body: Explorations into the Further Evolution of Human Nature*. Tarcher, 1993.

A wide-ranging look into transcending the limits of functional movement and the practices that historically have been used to achieve extraordinary human performance.

Netter, Frank H. *Atlas of Human Anatomy*, 6th ed. Saunders, 2014

One of the foundational elements of moving better as a runner is gaining an awareness of the musculoskeletal system. Netter's book provides the reader with a working vocabulary of human anatomy.

Noakes, Dr. Tim. *Lore of Running*, 4th ed. Human Kinetics, 2002

This tome covers nearly every topic you can imagine related to training and the history, biology, and psychology of running. Noakes applies both his ultrarunning experience and his research skills to sharing his understanding of the sport.

Raiport, Grigori. *Red Gold: Performance Techniques of the Russian and East German Olympic Victors*. Tarcher, 1988.

The Soviet sports machine was on the cutting edge not only of physical training techniques but also of psychological training. Raiport digs into the art and science of the approach to training the body and mind that fueled Soviet champions.

Romanov, Dr. Nicholas, with John Robson. *Dr. Nicholas Romanov's Pose Method of Running*. Pose Tech Press, 2004.

Olympic coach and sports scientist Romanov presents his philosophy and method for teaching the perfect running form seen in world-class runners. Romanov explains how to work with gravity in terms of positions (or poses) and how to move between those positions. The book includes drills and stretching and strengthening exercises.

Verkhoshansky, Yuri. *Supertraining*, 6th ed. Self-published, 2009.

A highly technical read, but worth it if you want a complete understanding of what's going on under the hood when you exercise and the adaptations your body makes to that exercise. Topics include overtraining, the impact of training on the immune system, and strategies on how to best use the adaptation process.

Wolf, Robb. *The Paleo Solution: The Original Human Diet*. Victory Belt Publishing, 2010.

Written for the layman by a former vegetarian. Wolf delves into the biochemistry of how poor diet choices can have adverse effects on digestion and overall health, with a thorough case being made for the Paleo diet. Includes recipes and an exercise section.

INDEX

ABOUT THE AUTHORS

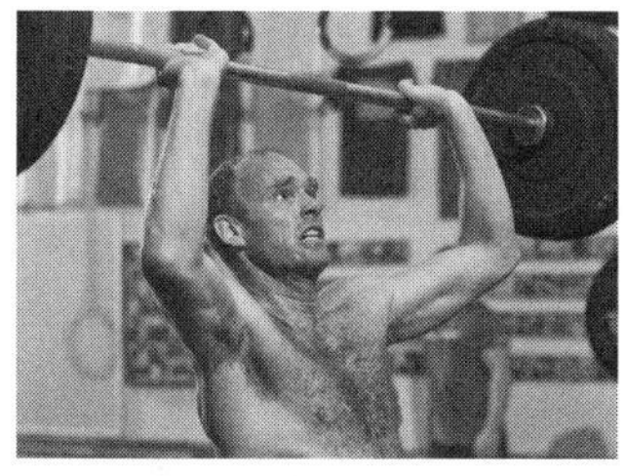

‹ T.J. MURPHY started his career in publishing as an assistant editor for *Triathlete* magazine in 1996. Before that, he held a series of odd jobs that turned out to be part of an education that he has since drawn upon: bike messenger, sports massage therapist, running shoe salesman, and unpaid assistant running coach for the Golden Gate Triathlon club. His magazine career has included stints as editor in chief for *Triathlete* magazine and *Inside Triathlon* and as editorial director of *Competitor* magazine. In 2012, he chronicled his personal odyssey into strength, conditioning, and mobility in his book *Inside the Box: How CrossFit Shredded the Rules, Stripped Down the Gym, and Rebuilt My Body.*

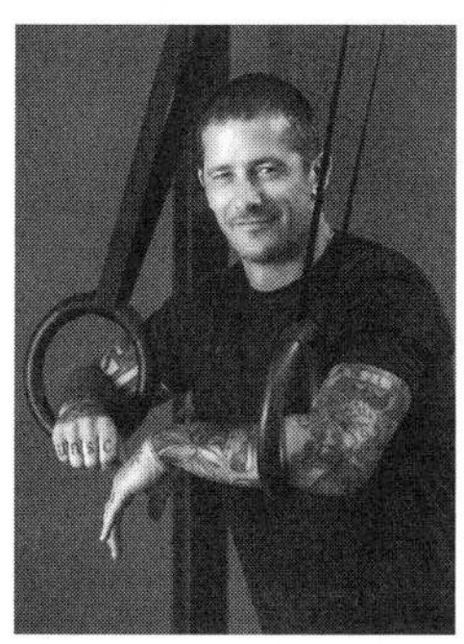

‹ BRIAN MACKENZIE is a world-renowned strength and conditioning coach and the innovator of the endurance/strength and conditioning paradigm. He is the author of

Power, Speed, ENDURANCE and creator of CrossFit Endurance (www.crossfitendurance.com), which specializes in movement with an emphasis on running, cycling, and swimming mechanics. MacKenzie and his program have been featured in *Competitor* magazine, *Runner's World*, *Triathlete* magazine, *Men's Journal*, *ESPN RISE* magazine, *The Economist*, Timothy Ferriss's *New York Times* best seller *The 4-Hour Body*, *Men's Running* UK, *Los Angeles Sports & Fitness* magazine, and *Riviera* magazine. MacKenzie has consulted with several teams, including the 2012 Western Athletic Conference Champions San Jose State Women's Swim Team, and worked with top athletes including Erin Cafaro (2-time Olympic gold medalist in women's 8+ rowing), Taylor Ritzel (Olympic gold medalist in women's 8+ rowing), Sara Hendershot (Olympian in women's pair rowing), Jamie Mitchell (10-time Molokai 2 Oahu Paddleboard champion), and Rich Froning (4-time CrossFit Games champion).